Kohlhammer

Versorgung gestalten – Gestaltung der Gesundheits- und Sozialversorgung heute und morgen

Herausgegeben von

Jürgen Zerth und Elmar Nass

Die Reihe „Versorgung gestalten" umfasst sowohl Monographien als auch Sammelbände, die das Themenfeld Gesundheitsversorgung aus interdisziplinärer Perspektive untersuchen.

Gesundheits- und Pflegeprozesse sind immer Beziehungen zwischen Ärzten, Patienten, Pflegenden und Gepflegten. Diese Beziehungen sind jedoch in einer organisatorischen und finanziellen Gestaltungsstruktur eingebettet, die wiederum integraler Bestandteil von (regulierten) Marktmechanismen ist. In diesem Sinne sind handlungstheoretische Perspektiven und Begründungsebenen genauso relevant wie die Auseinandersetzung mit organisationstheoretischen Anreiz- und Managementaspekten sowie werteorientierten Führungs- und Leitungsstrukturen. Die Reihe greift daher Fragestellungen der Handlungs- wie Organisationsebene im Gesundheitswesen genauso auf wie Aspekte der Technologieimplementierung im Gesundheits- und Sozialmarkt und den damit einhergehenden Konsequenzen für Akteure, Betroffene, Organisationen und Institutionen.

Die Analyse übergeordneter institutioneller Strukturen (regulierter) Gesundheitsmärkte komplettiert den interdisziplinären Blick auf die Herausforderung „Versorgung gestalten".

Jan Schildmann/Charlotte Buch/Jürgen Zerth (Eds.)

Defining the Value of Medical Interventions

Normative and Empirical Challenges

Verlag W. Kohlhammer

1. Auflage 2021

Alle Rechte vorbehalten
© W. Kohlhammer GmbH, Stuttgart
Gesamtherstellung: W. Kohlhammer GmbH, Stuttgart
Satz: Andrea Töcker, Neuendettelsau

Print:
ISBN 978-3-17-038176-6

E-Book-Format:
pdf: ISBN 978-3-17-038177-3

Für den Inhalt abgedruckter oder verlinkter Websites ist ausschließlich der jeweilige Betreiber verantwortlich. Die W. Kohlhammer GmbH hat keinen Einfluss auf die verknüpften Seiten und übernimmt hierfür keinerlei Haftung.

Table of contents

Value(s) in healthcare.
Introduction and theoretical premises

Jan Schildmann / Charlotte Buch / Jürgen Zerth
Defining the value of medical interventions – a brief introduction 9

Francisca Stutzin Donoso
The concepts of 'health' and 'disease'
Underlying assumptions in the idea of value in medical interventions ... 15

Karla Alex
Ethical conceptualization of a sustainable right to health(care) 29

Value(s) in healthcare.
Interdisciplinary Analyses

Paul Mark Mitchell
The cost-effectiveness of what in health and care? 51

Jasper Ubels
The assessment of value in health economics: utility and capability 69

Sebastian Himmler
Estimating the monetary value of health: why and how 83

Charlotte Buch / Jan Schildmann / Jürgen Zerth
Risk-sharing schemes to finance expensive pharmaceuticals
Interdisciplinary analyses 99

Including values and preferences by patients in healthcare.
Methods and case studies

Caroline Steigenberger / Petra Schnell-Inderst / Uwe Siebert
Integrating patients and social aspects into health
technology assessment 115

Karolina Napiwodzka
The shared decision-making model and practical discourse to foster
the appreciation of patients' value preferences in Polish healthcare 135

Jordan A. Parsons
Death or dialysis: the value of burdensome life-extending treatments
for the cognitively impaired 157

Contributors 175

Value(s) in healthcare.
Introduction and theoretical premises

Defining the value of medical interventions – a brief introduction

Discussions of how to define the value of medical interventions and the impacts concerning societal consequences have gained considerable attention during the last few decades. Different factors should be mentioned regarding that development. Firstly, a rectangularization of survival curve depicts the important impacts of a so-called demographic change in all industrialised countries. Not only have the proportions of elderly patients become more dominant, but the development of medical progress opens up new possibilities for diagnosis and treatment. Consequently, the so-called demographic effect can be explained endogenously by different factors which help patients to live longer and with a higher quality of life. Secondly, the progress of medical technologies reopens the discussion on the upper bounds a solidarity-based healthcare system is willing to bear. Finally, several new drugs and other interventions coming at high costs have been developed and approved in recent years. In Germany, for example the costs for anti-cancer drugs in 2017 were almost 6 billion EUR of around 38 billion spent on drugs by the statutory health insurance. Costs for anti-cancer drugs increased by more than 15 per cent compared to 2016.

Given the limited solidarity-based budget and the drivers of expenditures in healthcare mentioned previously, there is little surprise that the calls for investigating the value of healthcare interventions and the overall value of health itself have become more pressing. In this context, the term *value-based healthcare* has been used increasingly in debates about cost outcomes and necessities of health interventions. *Value* here refers to the regard we ascribe to something or the worth we think something should deserve. The US-American economist Michael Porter described the focus and goal of value-based healthcare in a contribution to the New England Journal of Medicine in 2009 as follows:

> The central focus must be on increasing value for patients – the health outcomes achieved per dollar spent. Good outcomes that are achieved efficiently are the goal, not the false 'savings' from cost shifting and restricted services. Indeed, the only way to truly contain costs in health care is to improve outcomes: in a value-based system, achieving and maintaining good health is inherently less costly than dealing with poor health.

Accordingly, *value*, as outlined above, refers to the quotient of costs and benefit of a health intervention. While Porter's account of value-based healthcare (or "value-based system" as in the title of the respective article) is directed at a series of changes proposed to reform the US healthcare system, the concept has been taken up by many proponents especially in the debate about the costs and benefits of cancer treatment.

However, the concept of *value* as proposed in the context of *value-based healthcare* is not the only possible understanding of the term. Value or values also describe principles according to which we judge what is important in life. In this respect, values are held on an individual level, but they can also be shared by a group of people and, at least, values should be a main column of organised, institutionalized healthcare services. These understandings of the term can obviously be linked but, at the same time, it is important to clarify what we refer to when talking about the value of medical interventions. With this book, we provide a collection of articles which take up different perspectives on the meaning of value in healthcare.

This book is the result of a process which took place over two years, during which junior researchers from a range of normative and empirical disciplines contributed to the topic of "defining the value of medical interventions". At the centre of this process was a conference at Wilhelm Löhe Hochschule in Fuerth, which took place in September 2019, near the ancient Franconian city of Nuremberg. The conference itself was based on the scientific workshop of the young scientists discussing their abstracts with each other combined with invited experts, reflecting the interdisciplinary approach. Moreover, some additional discourses took place in a broader sense. Two invited representatives of IQWiG (Institute for Quality and Efficiency in Health Care), Naomi Fujita-Rohwerder and Katharina Wölke, gave different insights into the German assessment strategy for valuating nondrug interventions and described the concept of early benefit assessment for pharmaceuticals. Michael Parker (University of Oxford) gave a short presentation on the first results of the Working Group "Research in global health emergencies". Some discussions on the necessity for an adequate implementation of beneficiaries of healthcare interventions occurred. In order to stress the role of different caregivers in health and social care markets, Jürgen Zerth (Wilhelm Loehe University of Applied Science) also discussed the need to rethink the role of social entrepreneurship regarding the linkage of organised healthcare, long-term care markets and different institutional approaches to cover social care needs. At the end of the conference week, a public discussion with different stakeholders from the German healthcare sector took place in Nuremberg in order to give forms of participation for the public.

The Scientific Conference

The preparations for the conference "Defining the value of medical interventions. Normative and empirical challenges" (funded by the German Federal

Ministry of Education and Research (01GP1883)) started with a call for abstracts, followed by a selection of contributions based on the scientific quality and scope of the papers, and our aim to further the discussion on recent developments and different disciplinary perspectives on defining the value of medical interventions. All the participants invited received personalised feedback on their abstracts and information on the contributions of the other participants. Those presentations that were connected thematically close were grouped together as part of the workshop programme. The conference offered a unique opportunity not only for presentations by all the participants but also plenty of time for discussion on each contribution. In addition, three workshops with the scientific and healthcare specialists mentioned above provided an opportunity for further in-depth discussions. Subsequently, all the participants were invited to submit a manuscript of their presentation, taking into account the feedback they had received at the conference. All manuscripts have been reviewed by at least one conference participant and one editor with a focus on the content of each chapter and links between the different contributions.

The contributions

1. Value(s) in healthcare. Introduction and theoretical premises

One fundamental challenge in the debate about the value of medical interventions (and also a much-discussed question at the conference) is to find a theoretical consensus about how to define value(s) in healthcare, which also means the value of health, hence medical interventions. Against the background of several theoretical approaches to this question, the contributions in the first part provide insights into theoretical premises for understanding value(s) in healthcare.

Francisca Stutzin Donoso's article *The concepts of 'health' and 'disease': underlying assumptions in the idea of value in medical interventions* provides an introduction into the debate, in so far as it discusses the fundamental concepts of health and disease, which is an indispensable background when talking about the value of medical interventions. Her article presents multiple existing definitions of health and disease and points out potential deficiencies and general criticisms. Based on her analysis, she provides an account of elements of disease concepts, which allow contextualisation of health outcomes and the value(s) of medical interventions.

Karla Alex discusses the connection between the right to health and healthcare and the concept of sustainability in *Ethical conceptualization of a sustainable right to health(care)*. Influenced by Thomas Nagel's defence of normative realisms, her line of argumentation starts with the objective instrumental value of health which follows from the objective intrinsic value of a human being. According to her subsequent analysis, a sustainable right to health(care) comprises an agent-relative and an agent-neutral right to health(care) and also tackles economic aspects. Furthermore, in the conceptualisation of a sustainable right to health, environmental aspects are encompassed.

2.   Value in healthcare. Interdisciplinary analyses

Defining the value of medical interventions is relevant for proceeding through the regulated benefit basket and what the different stakeholders in the regulated healthcare markets face regarding the reimbursement process. The value assigned determines the monetary equivalent an individual or society is willing to pay for the intervention. However, without a standardised definition of what value is, the development of methodologies to assess the value of certain medical interventions is not an easy task. Multiple approaches exist at the macro level, and they differ a lot across different health systems depending on the political and legal framework and institutional characteristics. Different approaches can differ on a micro level even within one system according to the respective needs, preferences and stakeholders included. Against this background, the second part of the publication comprises contributions covering exemplary value assessments and financing approaches and their health economical and interdisciplinary analyses.

Paul Mark Mitchell starts with the presentation of the well-known quality-adjusted life years (QALYs) approach as a health-economical way of defining value in healthcare in his article *The cost-effectiveness of what in health and care?*. The author analyses the criticism of this approach in his work and introduces the evaluation of people's capabilities as an alternative approach to inform health and care decision-making. According to his analysis, shifting to a "sufficient capability" objective may help to address efficiency and equity concerns related to decisions about the value of medical interventions

Jasper Ubels provides an analysis which links well to the preceding chapter by taking up the introduced concepts of QALY and the capability approach in *The assessment of value in health economics: utility and capability*. Subsequent to a reflection of the multiple conceptualisations of utility and a critique of both QALY and the capability approach, he argues for a combined measure of the value of medical interventions which includes information about capability, functioning and utility.

Sebastian Himmler's article *Estimating the monetary value of health: why and how* presents a justification of why assigning a monetary value to health (QALY) is necessary and different methodologies to estimate such a value. The author outlines an alternative approach in his contribution for estimating the monetary societal valuation of a QALY: the well-being valuation approach. In addition, the author presents first results of applying this approach in two different contexts and provides an analysis of the methodological limits of the approach presented.

Charlotte Buch, Jan Schildmann and **Jürgen Zerth** address the risks for both the payer and the pharmaceutical company in terms of real-world effectiveness and, subsequently, financial predictability in their article *Risk-sharing schemes to finance expensive pharmaceuticals. Interdisciplinary analyses.* Value-based pricing is described as a possible approach to control pharmaceutical expenditures, whereby on a micro-perspective level, this is employed as risk-sharing agreements (either financial- or performance-based) between payers and pharmaceutical companies. The article provides a theoretical account and a case study of performance-based risk-sharing agreements.

3. Including values and preferences by patients in healthcare. Methods and case studies

An important, nevertheless, sometimes underestimated perspective when defining the value of medical interventions is the implementation of patients' views, hence their values and preferences. As a "user" of medical interventions, however physician-induced, the patients are usually also the direct or indirect payer for healthcare. Patients are eventually the reason for all efforts regarding, for example, the definition of values, subsequent remunerations according to the value and fostering of continuous innovations. Therefore, the final part of this book focuses on the patients' perspective on an individual and societal level.

Caroline Steigenberger, Petra Schnell-Inderst and **Uwe Siebert** analyse how the perspective of patients and the social perspective can be included in Health Technology Assessments (HTAs) in their article *Integrating patients and social aspects into health technology assessment.* The authors argue that such an integrative approach is highly relevant in order to understand the needs, values and preferences of the users of a medical intervention. In the light of lacking implementation, the authors present an approach to systematically elaborate the patients' and social aspects within HTA taking the example of an HTA on integrative mistletoe therapy for patients with breast cancer.

Karolina Napiwodzka emphasises the importance of participatory decision-making for the eliciting of values on the micro-level in her article *The shared decision-making model and practical discourse to foster the appreciation of patients' value preferences in Polish healthcare. Discussing potentials and challenges.* In her contribution, which places the Polish healthcare system at the centre of her investigation, she analyses cognitive and communicative skills, active engagement and participation as premises for the shared understanding of values and respective responsibilities.

The part and book concludes with a contribution by **Jordan A. Parsons** on *Death or dialysis: The value of burdensome life-extending treatments for the cognitively impaired.* Taking the example of decision-making about dialysis, he analyses the factors relevant for the evaluation of the burdens and benefits of the interventions with a focus on situations in which treatment may be ended. The evaluation of benefit and harm of life-sustaining treatment is usually based on the subject's perceptions and views. In his analysis, the author focuses on decisions in the particularly challenging cases of patients who are not able to communicate their preferences and values due to a lack of decisional capacity.

The brief outline above indicates that this book offers not only a wide range of topics but also disciplinary perspectives on the different facets of the value of medical interventions and reflects a guided interdisciplinary approach for discussion and induced political advice.

The editors hope that this book provides interesting multi- and, in parts, interdisciplinary perspectives on the value of medical interventions and related values. We are very grateful to all the authors for their articles and their willingness to contribute to this volume. We would like to thank Philip Saunders for proofreading and the Peter-Oberender-Stiftung for the support of a professional formatting service. Additionally, we gratefully thank Anna-Kathleen Piereth for different assistance during the conference. Finally, we thank the German Federal Ministry of Education and Research for funding the conference and this publication.

Halle (Saale) and Fuerth, December 2020

Jan Schildmann, Charlotte Buch, Jürgen Zerth

The concepts of 'health' and 'disease'

Underlying assumptions in the idea of value in medical interventions

Francisca Stutzin Donoso

Abstract

This chapter provides an overview of the problem of conceptual definition of 'health' and 'disease' as a background to situate and introduce the discussion about health outcomes and value of new medical interventions. This work reflects and discusses broader literature on this topic by highlighting the available – and lacking – definitions in the specific context of health institutions in the UK. After introducing the World Health Organization's (WHO) definition of 'health' and some general criticisms of it, two more recent and particularly relevant positive definitions of 'health' are presented, stressing the potential connection between such definitions and the role of healthcare services. This is followed by a more extensive analysis of positive definitions of 'disease' since the technical literature seems particularly prolific and relevant. In order to organise the discussion, this chapter frames the different approaches to positive definitions of 'disease' within the fact/value problem. At the same time that it introduces three of the most influential conceptualisations of disease (Biostatistical Theory, The APA Task Force work and the Harm Dysfunction Analysis), it illustrates three possible positions regarding the fact/value problem in this matter (strong descriptivism, strong normativism, and mixed descriptive/normativism, respectively). Finally, because of the lack of a successful and agreed definition of 'disease', this chapter highlights recent efforts to embrace the disjunctive and vague elements of this concept, allowing and encouraging specific and contextual cluster definitions of 'disease', which seem particularly useful to contextualise and open the discussion on how to think about the idea of health outcomes and value in medical interventions.

Keywords: philosophy of medicine, concept of 'health', concept of 'disease', line-drawing problem, contextual definitions, goals of medicine

1 Introduction: building the bridge between the concepts of 'health' and 'disease' and the of idea value in medical interventions

Conceptual constructs tend to become naturalised and their meanings are taken for granted in the work to push disciplines further. Although this might be necessary to some extent, keeping in mind the frailty of conceptual definitions may be just as important for disciplines to move forward without oversimplifying or lacking context and complexity. Thus, by taking a step back and focusing on the question of what *is* value in the context of new medical interventions, this book highlights the importance of conceptual discussions in the background of highly applied fields associated with healthcare delivery which face challenging practical decisions of prioritisation, resource allocation and conflicting goals.

Although this is an issue of rich discussion – further explored in other chapters of this book – 'value' in healthcare is understood in general terms as patient health outcomes achieved per money spent, and so, it is argued to encompass many healthcare goals (Porter, 2010). However, the idea of health outcomes itself is a huge topic of discussion and this way of operationalising health, although needed, also faces significant challenges, not just on how to define them, but also how to measure them. In the specific context of the United Kingdom (UK), the National Health Service (NHS) has developed an outcomes framework to measure institutional progress. The framework is organised around five key dimensions:

- preventing people from dying prematurely
- enhancing the quality of life for people with long-term conditions
- helping people to recover from episodes of ill health or following injury
- ensuring that people have a positive experience of care
- treating and caring for people in a safe environment and protecting them from avoidable harm (NHS, 2020).

Although analysing these dimensions in-depth goes beyond the scope of this work, acknowledging this framework serves the purpose of showing how sanitary goals and health outcomes can potentially raise tensions when prioritising.

It is clearly unfeasible to pursue all these outcomes simultaneously and some may come into direct conflict with one another. A good example of this is how sometimes enhancing the quality of life of someone living with a long-term condition may imply that it is not possible to prevent that person from dying prematurely.[1]

---

[1] Parsons' contribution in this book discusses this precisely. The author argues that all patients (including those who lack decision-making capacity) ought to sometimes forego dialysis in favour of conservative kidney management, prioritising their quality of life over life-extending treatment.

Complexities associated with this are in direct connection with their immediate conceptual context, i.e. the concepts of 'health' and 'disease' to which this chapter is dedicated. Academic discussion around these two underlying concepts in all health-related issues is highly prolific and still unresolved. Usually taken for granted, one could claim these concepts may be central to defining when, how and with which goals medical interventions should be developed and applied, framing and contributing to the overarching focus of this book: exploring different definitions and approaches to value and how to incorporate these into the assessment of new medical interventions.

This chapter will argue that there needs to be a clear rationale connecting the concepts of 'health' (and 'disease'), health outcomes and the value of medical interventions to have consistent systems with clear and achievable goals in which results or measurements can actually be put into context and offer valuable input. We will see how this core idea underlies most of the problems presented in this book.[2]

The concepts of 'health' and 'disease' play an important part in everyone's daily experience of being alive and still manage to escape the descriptive possibilities of language – puzzling philosophers of science, sociologists, psychologists and many others, these concepts somehow invite Augustine's reflection on the question of "what, then, is time?" – so sensibly highlighted by Ricoeur in the preface to *Time and Narrative*, "I know well enough what it is, provided that nobody asks me; but if I am asked what it is and I try to explain, I am baffled" (Saint Augustin in Ricoeur, 1984, p. xi). Very similarly, addressing the concepts of 'health' and 'disease' implies engaging in an ongoing quest.

---

[2] Chapters in this book, which refer to this conceptual consistency issue, are those by Buch *et al.* on highly-priced pharmaceuticals and by Steigenberger *et al.* on integrating patients' and social aspects into Health Technology Assessments. In the first case, assessing whether certain pharmaceuticals are too expensive will depend heavily on what societies are willing to pay and this, in turn, might be argued to depend greatly on what the states of health and disease are. This latter point also applies to the second case, which focuses on patients' perceived value of the quality and benefit of a health technology.
More contributions in this book focused on economics, such as those by Himmler and Mitchell, exemplify and refer to this matter. These works use specific understandings and frameworks for the monetary value of health in terms of well-being, for example, those defined by a specific measurement of quality of life (quality-adjusted life years) (Himmler, in this volume). Mitchell's work (in this volume) challenges this notion, as the quality of life captured by quality-adjusted life years might be considered too narrow, suggesting a shift from outcomes focused on health (such as quality-adjusted life years) towards people's capabilities.

2 The complexities behind conceptualising health: Its operationalisation and the goals of medicine

The current Constitution of the NHS in the UK, last updated in 2015, does not define what counts as health or disease. However, it does state that the NHS' aims to improve health and well-being, supporting people to keep mentally and physically well, to help them get better when they are ill and, if they cannot fully recover, help them to stay as well as possible till the end of their lives (NHS, 2015). It is possible to see from this statement that the core idea underlying the use of the concept of 'health' mirrors a positive definition[3] based on a state of well-being that includes both a mental and physical dimension. The UK's National Institute for Health and Care Excellence (NICE) does not define health specifically but health-related quality of life as "a combination of a person's physical, mental and social well-being; not merely the absence of disease" (NICE, 2018). The NICE definition paraphrases one stated in and enforced by the WHO Constitution, according to which, "health is a state of complete physical, mental and social wellbeing and not merely the absence of disease or infirmity" (WHO, 1948). In this manner, the UK seems to embrace a positive understanding of health, rejecting negative definitions based on the absence of disease.

The *overall* assessment of the definition offered by the WHO proposes that by suggesting a positive operationalisation of the concept of 'health', it represents an improvement over previous negative definitions, but it, nonetheless, raises significant problems. These are mostly related to the idea of "complete well-being", which NICE omits.

Critical views on the definition offered by the WHO raise issues particularly relevant for the topic of this book. Some critiques suggest that it seems idealistic and unachievable, labelling most of the population as unhealthy most of the time. Critiques argue that this definition could contribute to the medicalisation of society, justify unlimited development of drugs or treatments, and create serious challenges for healthcare systems that have to find a balance between individual health needs and the resources available. Further critiques of this definition are related to disease patterns shifting from acute to chronic conditions, supporting the idea that conceptualisations of health and disease might be closely related to historical context and associated health developments. Additional critiques of this definition include, among many others, problems for disease classifications systems (e.g. quality of life, disability, functioning)

---

[3] In general terms, this means a definition focused on what health is instead of what it is not. Health defined as the absence of disease, for example, is usually described as a negative definition of health.

since health, as "complete" well-being, does not allow for measurement or operational specification (Bircher, 2005; Huber *et al.*, 2011).

In all critiques, these considerations work to bridge the gap between the relevant conceptualisations of health and disease and define the value of medical interventions. Broadly speaking, if the value of medical interventions comes from a focus on improving the health and reducing the disease burden on individuals and populations, then what counts as 'health' and 'disease' matters.

Although there is still no consensus on a satisfactory positive definition of the concept of 'health', or even on whether this is possible or desirable (Boorse, 2011), many interesting new definitions have arisen from the discussion. I will introduce two rather recent positive definitions of health that serve the purpose of illustrating a broader and more nuanced view on this issue, stimulating insightful reflection for this particular work. Bircher (2005) suggests conceptualising health as,

> a dynamic state of wellbeing characterized by a physical, mental and social potential, which satisfies the demands of a life commensurate with age, culture, and personal responsibility. If the potential is insufficient to satisfy these demands the state is disease. (Bircher, 2005, p. 336)

This definition seems to be an overall improvement of the definition offered by the WHO because it allows health to be a variable state within the lifespan of an individual, attending to relevant dimensions and being, in this sense, more realistic. However, this definition resorts to controversial or difficult concepts – mental and social potential and personal responsibility – that would also require a definition for this concept of 'health' to be practicable.

In contrast to this long-winded definition, Huber *et al.* (2011, p. 2) define health as the "ability to adapt and self-manage", with specific characterisations in the three domains of health: physical, mental and social. This understanding of health seems particularly interesting because it diverges completely from the WHO legacy, stressing the capacity or functioning of the individual, thus, potentially reconfiguring the role of healthcare services and the value of medical interventions in terms of support towards developing such functioning.

Furthermore, this definition may be particularly relevant in current times when chronic diseases are the main disease burden in the UK and the rest of the world. Chronic diseases currently account for 90 % of all deaths in the UK, and the risk of dying prematurely from a chronic disease is 11 % (Office for National Statistics, 2017; WHO, 2017).[4] Furthermore, chronic diseases account for 50 % of all general practice appointments, 64 % of outpatient appointments, 70 % of all inpatient bed days and 70 % of the total health and care expenditure

---

[4]   These statistics are based on the four main groups of non-communicable chronic diseases (cardiovascular disease, cancer, diabetes and obstructive pulmonary disease).

in England (Department of Health, 2012).[5] This information implies that currently and in terms of disease burden, full recovery is not an option in most cases, therefore, self-management and the possibility to mobilise resources become key concepts in assessing the value of medical interventions (Bodenheimer *et al.*, 2002). This idea of self-management and the possibility to mobilise resources remains closely linked to the capabilities approach and its application to this field.[6]

3   The complexities behind conceptualising disease: what can we learn from key definitions?

Regarding positive definitions of 'disease', those that do not merely place explanatory value on the absence of health, the overall picture is just as dynamic and unresolved. This discussion is very prolific both in terms of the literature generated and the many working definitions (Lemoine, 2013; Walker and Rogers, 2018). However, specifically in the context of official health institutions in the UK, neither the NHS nor NICE acknowledges or defines of the concept of 'disease' or any other related concepts such as 'disorder', 'condition', 'sickness', 'infirmity' or 'illness'. Therefore, it might be thought that such national institutions implicitly embrace a negative definition of 'disease' by setting their focus on health. In other words, 'disease' is broadly taken to be the absence of health.

As an effort to systematise the extensive literature on the concept of 'disease', Boorse (2011) suggests that there are five commonly present elements in most 'health' and 'disease' definitions. These elements include (1) medical treatment, (2) pain, discomfort and disability, (3) statistical abnormality, (4) disvalue and (5) specific biological ideas: homeostasis, fitness and adaptation. However, counter-examples for each of these elements show that all fail to be neither necessary nor sufficient for a satisfactory definition of these concepts at an abstract theoretical level,[7] thus, illustrating how challenging it seems to be to reach satisfactory definitions.

---

[5]   These statistics are based on a category of chronic diseases that is not restricted to non-communicable diseases, though it includes the main four groups as well (cardiovascular disease, cancer, diabetes and obstructive pulmonary disease).

[6]   This is discussed in-depth later in this bood in the chapters by Mitchell – briefly mentioned previously – and Ubels, who highlights the importance of combining information about capability, functioning and utility in the assessment of the value of medical interventions.

[7]   Counter-examples for each element include (1) all disease for which there is no treatment available and, conversely, non-disease medical treatments, such as plastic surgery or contraceptive pills; (2) pathological conditions that do not involve pain, discomfort or disability, such as hypertension, and, conversely, non-pathological conditions that may involve all or some of these elements, such as pregnancy; (3) many statistically abnormal

Traditional conceptual analysis in philosophy broadly implies aiming at an exact, descriptive definition by "testing a definitional criteria and exceptions against a set of given cases, while drawing up counter-cases against an opponent's definition", thus, identifying conditions that are both necessary and sufficient to define a concept and the exceptions to these conditions (Lemoine, 2013, p. 310). However, because of the lack of a satisfactory descriptive definition of 'health' and 'disease', it has been argued that conceptual analysis can provide *descriptive* or *naturalist* (factual) definitions or *normativist* (value) definitions. The former are value-free definitional criteria, while the latter are value-laden definitional criteria, broadly assuming that disease is bad for the person and health is desirable. Although most authors provide some kind of normativist definitional criteria for 'health' and 'disease', which may be soft, in the sense that may also include some descriptive conditions, some very influential definitions adopt a strong descriptive approach, stressing the importance to continue working on value-free definitional criteria for 'health' and 'disease' (Boorse, 2011; Lemoine, 2013).

In order to illustrate this very dynamic discussion and provide some background on what is the state-of-the-art, it seems relevant to present some of the most influential definitions of the concept of 'disease'. These include Boorse's (1977) Biostatistical Theory, which represents a strong descriptivist (value-free) position, Spitzer and Endicott's (1978) tentative proposed definition and criteria of medical and mental disorder, which represents a rather normativist (value-laden) position, and Wakefield's (1992) Harm Dysfunction Analysis, which represents a mixed position, stressing the importance of naturalist and normativist components.

Boorse's (1977) *Biostatistical Theory*, being largely laden towards normativist definitions of 'health' and 'disease', emerges as a strong critique of previous literature on the topic. The author offers a strong descriptive definition, stressing that health and disease evaluations are sensitive to contextual and indivi-

---

conditions are not diseases, such as being left-handed and, conversely, many statistically normal conditions involve a pathological condition such as gum disease or tooth decay; and (4) depending on the context, a disease may not necessarily be bad for the individual. An example of this would be that flat feet during a period of war might save someone's life by precluding them from joining the armed forces, thus, potentially being regarded as a good thing. Finally, (5) many non-disease human functions are not homeostatic, such as growth or reproduction, and, conversely, pathologies such as sterility do not produce any homeostatic failure. If one considers that fitness stands for individual survival and reproduction, many pathological conditions do not interfere with these, such as anosmia, and, conversely, many non-pathological activities, such as mountaineering, may increase the risk of early death. Regarding adaptation, depending on the context, some diseases may not be maladaptive. An example of this would be a severe immune deficiency in a sterile environment (plastic bubble) and, conversely, many non-pathological conditions may be adaptive in one context and not in another, such as being light-skinned in Iceland or in Africa (Boorse, 2011).

dual variables, highlighting that the conceptual definition should be value-free to allow the individual to value the condition according to relevant specific circumstances. In this manner, according to the *Biostatistical Theory*, 'health' is defined by normal functioning, where what is normal is statistically determined and functioning refers to biological functions. Furthermore, 'disease' consists of deviations from the species' biological design, therefore, identifying 'disease' is considered a matter of natural sciences rather than an evaluative judgment. Thus, the overall rationale and assumptions underlying this definition imply four main criteria: (1) definition of the reference class (an age group of a sex of a species), (2) definition of normal function within members (based on a statistically typical contribution to the individual survival and reproduction), (3) definition of 'health' in a member of the reference class as a normal functional ability and (4) definition of 'disease' as an internal state which reduces functional abilities below typical efficiency (Boorse, 1977).

Spitzer and Endicott (1978), building on their previous work as members of the American Psychiatric Association Task Force on Nomenclature and Statistics (which suggested a largely criticised first definition of the concept of medical and mental disorder in 1976), provide a revised definition of these concepts, which states that,

> a medical disorder is a relatively distinct condition resulting from an organismic dysfunction, which in its fully developed or extreme form is directly and intrinsically associated with distress, disability, or certain other types of disadvantage. The disadvantage may be of a physical, perceptual, sexual, or interpersonal nature. Implicitly there is a call for action on the part of the person who has the condition, the medical or its allied professions, and society. A mental disorder is a medical disorder whose manifestations are primarily signs or symptoms of psychological (behavioural) nature, or if physical, can be understood only using psychological concepts. (Spitzer and Endicott, 1978, p. 18)

Thus, this definition comprises three fundamental ideas within the notion of medical disorder, which altogether convey the overall message that something has gone wrong in the human organism. This gives special importance to the evaluative aspect of the concept: (1) negative consequences of the condition, (2) an inferred or identified organismic dysfunction, and (3) an implicit call for action to the medical profession, the person with the condition and the society in terms of granting exemptions from certain responsibilities to those in the sick role, as well as providing a means for delivery of medical care (Spitzer and Endicott, 1978). It is important to note that these authors' ultimate interest is to define the concept of 'mental disorder', and since they decide to do this by considering it a subgenre of medical disorders, they also provide a definition of 'medical disorder'. However, because of this ultimate interest, the definition avoids using the word 'disease' as, according to these authors, it generally denotes a progressive physical disorder of known physiopathology, which is not the case for most mental disorders. Therefore, the concept of organismic dysfunction, or its negative consequences, do not imply that these have a physical nature (Spitzer and Endicott, 1978). Although analysing this definition further goes beyond the interest of this revision, it is worth noting that the authors add a list of four criteria which, they argue, must be met in order for a condition to be classified as a disorder.

Wakefield's (1992) Harm Dysfunction Analysis emerges from a detailed critical analysis of several accounts, including that of Boorse (1977) and Spitzer and Endicott (1978). This author's main point is that a definition of the concept of disorder requires both an evaluation (normativist) based on social norms and a scientific (descriptive) understanding of the failure of physical or mental mechanisms to perform natural functions as designed by evolution. Thus, according to Wakefield,

> a condition is a disorder if and only if (a) the condition causes harm or deprivation of benefit to the person as judged by the standards of the person's culture (the value criterion), and (b) the condition results from the inability of some internal mechanisms to perform its natural function, wherein a natural function is an effect that is part of the evolutionary explanation of the existence and structure of the mechanism (the explanatory criterion). (1992, p. 384)

For Wakefield, what follows then is a definition of mental disorders as a special case, where the nature of the cause of the symptoms determines a disorder as mental and not the nature of the symptom themselves.[8] Therefore,

> a condition is a mental disorder if and only if (a) the condition causes harm or deprivation of benefit to the person as judged by the standards of the person's culture (the value criterion), and (b) the condition results from the inability of some mental mechanisms to perform its natural function, wherein a natural function is an effect that is part of the evolutionary explanation of the existence and structure of the mental mechanism (the explanatory criterion). (Wakefield, 1992, p. 385)

However, as stated by this author, even the clearest concepts pose areas of vagueness and ambiguity, and, in this particular definition, this indeterminacy rests on how to distinguish mental from physical mechanisms (Wakefield, 1992).

All these working definitions of the concept of 'disease' share the idea that there is a discontinuity between health and disease, i.e. health and disease can be either present or absent. Nonetheless, the concept of dysfunction – that all these definitions share – admits different degrees and, therefore, raises the problem of using a continuous variable (dysfunction) as the basis for a catego-

---

[8]   This means that what is causing the symptom arises from a mental dysfunction and not that the symptom is mental dysfunction. Some symptoms, such as pain, are argued to be a mental phenomenon, but somatic dysfunctions may be the cause of pain, in which case, pain is not a mental disorder. Therefore, what matters regarding labelling purposes is that the nature of the cause of the symptom is mental.

rical definition.[9] This has been described as the line-drawing problem in 'disease' definition (Rogers and Walker, 2017b).

Building on various disease examples (cancer, UTI, TB), Rogers and Walker (2017b) argue that the more the scientific community learns about what constitutes 'disease', the more difficult it is to determine the relevant dysfunction associated with a condition. As such, the absolute philosophical perspective on disease does not reflect everyday medical practice with borderline cases, drawing boundaries as necessary for decision-making and practical purposes. So, according to Walker and Rogers (2018), the concept of 'disease' does not seem to be classically structured since it fails to be defined in classical ways (conceptual analysis leading to exact necessary and sufficient conditions). Following from this, the authors suggest that this concept should be approached as a disjunctive and vague concept, therefore, encouraging the academic community to focus on developing specific and contextual cluster definitions for specific reasons or aims (Walker and Rogers, 2018).[10]

4 Conclusion: embracing complexity

By briefly revising and discussing some key approaches to the concepts of 'health' and 'disease', the indeterminateness of both concepts becomes clear, suggesting that a reflexive and open perspective towards possible specific and contextual definitions that can respond to the needs of specific quests is adopted. It also becomes clear that health outcomes and, thus, the value of a new medical intervention, will vary accordingly that depending on the conceptualisation of 'health' and 'disease'. In this way, not only defining the value but also what *is* 'value' would require a contextual approach (for specific reasons or aims) that is consistent with conceptualisations of 'health' and 'disease'. If, in the context of the current predominance of chronic or long-term diseases, for example, one adopts the definition of 'health' as the ability to adapt and self-manage (Huber *et al.*, 2011), this would introduce a radical shift in how we conceive health outcomes and, thus, how we frame the value of new medical interventions.[11] However, I will briefly draw on Walker's (2019) ethical reflections about long-term treatment to reflect further on the shift introduced by contex-

---

[9] "Biological functions may categorically cease altogether (the heart may stop beating, the liver stop metabolising, and the kidneys stop filtering blood), but short of absolute cessation of function, there are degrees of performance all the way up to abundantly healthy levels" (Rogers and Walker, 2017b, p. 415).

[10] An example of such cluster definitions is Roger and Walker's (2017a, p. 277) working definition of borderline diseases as "X is a disease$_{ODx}$ if there is a dysfunction that has significant risk of causing severe harm".

[11] Parsons' chapter in this publication on quality of life and life-extending treatments is a good example of this.

tual definitions for specific aims. This author argues that long-term treatment can bring the principles of patients' beneficence and autonomy into tension. Therefore, although the treatment may benefit the patient's state of health, it might, simultaneously, hamper their autonomy by preventing them from doing things that are also important to them. In this way, health and other valuable aspects of life can come into conflict and, thus, healthcare professionals, in the specific context of long-term conditions, should do more than prescribe the best treatment available and enable patients to adhere (Walker, 2019).

> They should, where they can, act to ensure that their patients do adhere. Sometimes they cannot do this. But even in that situation there is often more they can do. They could, for example, switch the patient onto a different treatment plan, one she is more likely to adhere to. This is not, however, likely to be the best option. While it may be better for the patient than doing nothing, if the original treatment was preferred at the choice stage it is unlikely to be as beneficial as bringing it about that the patient adheres. (Walker, 2019, p. 141)

In this way, the goal of long-term treatment would focus on allowing patients to adhere even if this means prescribing a less effective treatment to which patients are more likely to adhere. This goal would be in line with an understanding of 'health' as the ability to adapt and self-manage (Huber *et al.*, 2011), potentially valuing a medical intervention to which patients are more likely to adhere over a more effective one to which patients are less likely to adhere.

As this example shows, these different focuses may also justify framing contextual definitions within different disciplines, trans-contextual or interdisciplinary perspectives, highlighting the relevance of embracing the inherent complexity of the matter. When it comes to social sciences' problems, such as those related to health and well-being, the existing categories and methods,

> will retain relevance only to the extent that they help us address real problems of these new disciplines. If they are of no discernible help, then it is best to ignore them for this case. (Alexandrova, 2015, p. 224)

This intrinsically flexible and contextual perspective may help us to understand and keep in mind the rigour required and the unavoidable complexity of working within the health sciences.[12] In this way, this book aims at embracing such complexity by comprising efforts from different disciplines and welco-

---

[12] Some especially interdisciplinary contributions in this book that exemplify this perspective include the work by Alex, which aims at integrating economic, social and ethical elements into the valuation of medical interventions, including the rights of future generations, and the work by Napiwodzka, which discusses the added value of patients' inclusion in clinical decision-making concerning diagnosis and treatment, with a strong focus on communication and discourse.

ming interdisciplinary works to address the question of what *is* value in the context of new medical interventions.

References

Alexandrova, A. (2015), "Well-being and Philosophy of Science", *Philosophy Compass*, Vol. 10 No. 3, pp. 219–231.

Bircher, J. (2005), "Towards a dynamic definition of health and disease", *Medicine, Health Care and Philosophy*, Vol. 8, pp. 335–341.

Bodenheimer, T., Wagner, E. and Grumbach, K. (2002), "Improving primary care for patients with chronic illness. The Chronic Care Model, Part 2", *Journal of the American Medical Association*, Vol. 288 No. 15, pp. 1909–1914.

Boorse, C. (1977), "Health as a theoretical concept", *Philosophy of Science*, Vol. 44 No. 4, pp. 542–573.

Boorse, C. (2011), "Concepts of Health and Disease", in Gifford, F. (Ed.), *Philosophy of Medicine (Handbook of the Philosophy of Science)*. Elsevier BV.

Department of Health (2012), *Long-term conditions compendium of information. Third edition*. Available at: https://www.gov.uk/government/publications/long-term-conditions-compendium-of-information-third-edition (accessed 2 December 2020).

Huber, M., Knottnerus, J. A., Green, L., van der Horst, H., Jadad, A. R., Kromhout, D., Leonard, B., Lorig, K., Loureiro, M. I., van der Meer, J. W. M., Schnabel, P., Smith, R., van Weel, C. and Smid, H. (2011), "How should we define health?", *British Medical Journal*, Vol. 343, pp. 1–3. doi: 10.1136/bmj.d4163.

Lemoine, M. (2013), "Defining disease beyond conceptual analysis: an analysis of conceptual analysis in philosophy of medicine", *Theoretical Medicine and Bioethics*, Vol. 34 No. 4, pp. 309–325.

NHS: National Health Service (2015), *The NHS Constitution for England - GOV.UK*. Available at: https://www.gov.uk/government/publications/the-nhs-constitution-for-england/the-nhs-constitution-for-england#patients-and-the-public-your-rights-and-the-nhs-pledges-to-you (accessed 2 December 2020).

NHS: National Health Service (2020), *About the NHS outcomes framework (NHS OF)*. Available at: https://digital.nhs.uk/data-and-information/publications/ci-hub/nhs-outcomes-framework#framework-domains (accessed 2 December 2020).

NICE (2018), *National Institute for Health and Care Excellence NICE*. Available at: https://www.nice.org.uk/glossary?letter=h (accessed 2 December 2020).

Office for National Statistics (2017), Avoidable mortality in England and Wales 2015. United Kingdom. Available at: https://www.ons.gov.uk/peoplepopulationandcommunity/healthandsocialcare/causesofdeath/bulletins/avoidablemortalityinenglandandwales/2015#things-you-need-to-know-about-this-release (accessed 2 December 2020).

Porter, M. (2010), "What is value in health care?", *The New England Journal of Medicine*, No. 363, pp. 2477–2481.

Ricoeur, P. (1984), *Time and narrative*. Translated by K. McLaughlin and D. Pellauer. Chicago and London: University of Chicago Press.

Rogers, W. and Walker, M. (2017a), "Defining disease in the context of overdiagnosis", *Medicine, Health Care and Philosophy*, Vol. 20, pp. 269–280. doi: 10.1007/s11019-016-9748-8.

Rogers, W. and Walker, M. (2017b), "The line-drawing problem in disease definition", *Journal of Medicine and Philosophy*, Vol. 42, pp. 405–423. doi: 10.1093/jmp/jhx010.

Spitzer, R. and Endicott, J. (1978), "Medical and mental disorder: proposed definition and criteria", in Klein, D. F. and Spitzer, R. L. (Eds.), *Critical issues in psychiatric diagnosis*. New York: Raven Press, pp. 15–39.

Wakefield, J. (1992), "The concept of mental disorder. On the boundary between biological facts and social values", *American Psychologist Association*, Vol. 47 No. 3, pp. 373–388.

Walker, M. and Rogers, W. (2018), "A new approach to defining disease", Journal of Medicine and Philosophy, Vol. 43, pp. 402–420. doi: 10.1093/jmp/jhy014.

Walker, T. (2019), *Ethics and chronic illness.* Routledge.

WHO: World Health Organization (1948), *Constitution of the World Health Organization.* Available at: http://apps.who.int/gb/bd/PDF/bd47/EN/constitution-en.pdf?ua=1 (accessed 2 December 2020).

WHO: World Health Organization (2017), *Noncommunicable diseases progress monitor 2017.* Geneva: World Health Organization.

Ethical conceptualization of a sustainable right to health(care)

Karla Alex

Abstract

Despite a vast amount of discussions on sustainability and on the right to health(care) within applied ethics, it has not been precisely determined how both concepts can be connected. This article argues that a sustainable right to health(care) comprises an agent-relative right to health(care), an agent-neutral right to health(care), economic aspects, and (only included in the conceptualization of a sustainable right to health, not to healthcare) environmental aspects. It starts with a formal outline of the argument in the form of numbered premises, with reference to the sections of the paper where the respective premises are analysed (section 1). It then summarises the idea that a sustainable right to health, encompassing the right to healthcare, rests on the assumptions of normative realism, of agent-relative and agent-neutral values (Nagel, 1986), and on the traditional concept of sustainability (Elkington, 1999) (sections 2 and 3). Concomitantly, the International Covenant on Economic, Social and Cultural Rights' (ICESCR, 1966) outline of the right to health and the World Commission on Environment and Development's (WCED, 1987) definition of sustainability are evaluated. Finally, the proposed concept is discussed from the perspective of different countries and with a focus on the conflict between economic and ethical, as well as agent-relative and agent-neutral aspects of a sustainable right to health(care) (section 4). Repeatedly in sections 3 and 4, germline genome editing is taken as an example for the suggested approach, as the health of future generations is, on the one hand, reflected in the idea of a sustainable right to health(care) and, on the other hand, is essential when discussing the right to this novel technology.

Keywords: agent-relative and agent-neutral value, right to health and right to healthcare, sustainability, future generations, germline genome editing

1   Outline of the argument

1.   From the value of health follows a universal right to health. (section 2.1 and 2.2)

2.   From the universality of the right to health follows a sustainable right to health. (section 3.1)

3.   The concept of sustainability originates in business ethics and traditionally comprises social aspects, economic aspects, and environmental aspects. (section 3.1)

4.   The value of health is both agent-neutral and agent-relative. Therefore, the universal right to health is agent-neutral as well as agent-relative. Therefore, the sustainable right to health is agent-neutral as well as agent-relative. (section 2.4; section 3.2)

5.   The agent-neutral sustainable right to health refers to the health of the entire, global society, at present and in future. (section 3.2)

6.   The agent-relative sustainable right to health refers to the health of any specific individual A in a specific situation. (section 3.2)

7.   The concept of a sustainable right to health comprises the traditional concept of sustainability as well as the health of any specific individual A in a specific situation as the agent-relative right to health. (section 3.2)

8.   The universal right to health encompasses the universal right to healthcare. (section 2.2)

9.   From the universality of the right to healthcare follows a sustainable right to healthcare. (section 3.1)

10. Because the sustainable right to health is agent-neutral as well as agent-relative, the sustainable right to healthcare is agent-neutral as well as agent-relative. (section 3.3)

11. The agent-neutral sustainable right to healthcare refers to the healthcare of the entire, global society, at present and in future. (section 3.3)

12. The agent-relative right to healthcare refers to the healthcare for any specific individual A in a specific situation, i.e. to any individual patient A. (section 3.3)

13. The concept of a sustainable right to healthcare does not comprise the environmental aspect of a sustainable right to health. The economic aspect is especially focusing on the health economy. The social aspect (agent-neutral right to healthcare) does not comprise the socio-economic components of the right to health. The concept of a sustainable right to healthcare, therefore, comprises the health of the individual patient (agent-relative right to healthcare), the health of each present and future member of society (agent-neutral right to healthcare), the economy of the healthcare system, not including economic interests that are beyond moral interests, i.e. none that exceed the guarantee of a sustainable right to healthcare. (section 3.3)

2   From the value of health follows a universal right to health and to healthcare

2.1 Objectivity of values (cf. Nagel, 1986)

In order to argue that the right to health follows from the existence of a value of health it first needs to be defined what is understood by value from the ethical perspective taken here. Following Thomas Nagel's chapter on "Value" in his book *The view from nowhere*, values are understood as to be grounded in "normative realism" (Nagel, 1986, p. 145) and to present reasons to act (cf. p. 138). As such, they are at least partially (cf. pp. 148f.) objective. Although Nagel does not prove normative realism but tries to defend it by refuting still refutable – e.g. his argument that to reduce pain is an objective value because it would "seem[] [...] insane" (p. 157) to assume that pain is merely a means to avoid painful, possibly life threatening situations, and not objectively valuable – objections to it (cf. p. 144), after all, from his perspective, it can be argued that there are at least any objective values (cf. pp. 148f.), and it might be argued that not the avoidance of pain, but the avoidance of death is objectively valua ble.

Nagel concludes normative realism from the assumption of "the possibility of realism" (p. 144). That is, the assumption that there is a reality that is not identical with "appearances" (p. 147). He argues that not merely physical reality but also normative reality can be described as a form of truth:

> Normative realism is the view that propositions about what gives us reasons for action can be true or false independently of how things appear to us, and that we can hope to discover the truth by transcending the appearances and subjecting them to critical assessment. What we aim to discover by this method is not a new aspect of the external world, called value, but rather just the truth about what we and others should do and want. (Nagel, 1986, p. 139)

Nagel would argue that health is an objective value because of his assumption of hedonism. However, there is another way to defend the objective normativity of health from the objectivity of values. Nagel considers whether there are intrinsic or, as he calls them, external values. Unlike all other values, these are not merely instrumental, i.e., a "value for anyone" (p. 153; emphasis in original). If there is an intrinsic value of an individual, such as a human being – as this article considers human health, the value of non-humans is not discussed, although, from an ethical perspective, it is, nevertheless, very important to consider non-anthropocentric conceptions of value, especially in discussions on the value of animal research for the development of new health technologies – it follows that there is a normative reason to generally preserve both the life and the health of human beings because of their intrinsic value. This rule notwithstanding, there might be exceptions to it in cases of end-of-life deci-sion-making (cf. Cummiskey, 2004), as "[r]easons may be universal [...] without forming a unified system that always provides a method for arriving at deter-minate conclusions about what one should do" (Nagel, 1986, p. 152).

From the objective intrinsic value of a human being, therefore, follows an objective instrumental value of health.

2.2 Definition of the right to health as encompassing socio-economic, environmental, and other rights and a right to healthcare (cf. ICESCR, 1966)

Like health, healthcare is of instrumental value (cf. DeCamp, 2019, p. 233; Por-ter, 2010, p. 2478) and results from the intrinsic value of the human being. The value of health and of healthcare is the normative basis for a right to health and to healthcare, as, in order to preserve the value of health and, thus, the intrinsic value of human beings, it is necessary to put this value into the legally binding form of a right, such as: "the right of everyone to the enjoyment of the highest attainable standard of physical and mental health" (ICESCR, 1966, Art. 12, para. 1). Throughout this paper, the shorter formulation 'right to health' can be understood as encompassing all aspects of this right as specified by the ICESCR in 1966 as well as in its *General Comment No. 14: The Right to the Highest Attainable Standard of Health (Art. 12)* by the United Nations' (UN) Committee on Economic, Social and Cultural Rights (CESCR, 2000).[1] Similarly, when I use the formulation 'right to healthcare', I refer to the specifications made in these international documents by the UN, as the right to health encompasses "the right to health care" (CESCR, 2000, para. 4). Furthermore, it encompasses socio-economic, environmental, and other rights, in detail:

> the right to health embraces a wide range of socio-economic factors that promote conditions in which people can lead a healthy life, and extends to the underlying determinants of health, such as food and nutrition, housing, access to safe and po-table water and adequate sanitation, safe and healthy working conditions, and a healthy environment. (CESCR, 2000, para. 4)

To grant the right to health to everyone, therefore, necessitates, on the one hand, the creation and sustaining of a healthy environment and healthy social conditions. On the other hand, it requires the provision of healthcare to every-one.

---

[1]   Cf. the preceding article by Stutzin Donoso in this volume for a discussion of the defini-tion of health.

2.3 Refutation of arguments against a universal right to healthcare

Because the right to health and to healthcare is guaranteed to everyone, it is called universal. In response to the definition of this universal right to healthcare by the ICESCR in 1966, some authors have argued that there is no right to healthcare. In the following, by referring to the *General Comment* (CESCR, 2000), I will try to refute several aspects of this line of argument as put forward in two selected articles on the issue (Baumrin, 2012; Narveson, 2011).

In his article "Why There Is No Right to Health Care", published in *Medicine and Social Justice: Essays on the Distribution of Health Care* (Rhodes *et al.*, 2012), Stefan Bernard Baumrin points out that as 'ought implies can', there can be no universal right to healthcare because it is impossible for any individual state to guarantee universal healthcare for the entire world: "no state thinks itself obliged, nor is it able to provide health care for everyone (i.e., of every nation)" (Baumrin, 2012, p. 93). This is the same argument presented by both Michael Green in "Global Justice and Health: Is Health Care a Basic Right" (cf. Green, 2004, p. 215) and Jan Narveson in "The Medical Minimum: Zero" (cf. Narveson, 2011, p. 563). It is an interesting objection and points to what the CESCR states in its comment on article 12: "The Committee is aware that, for millions of people throughout the world, the full enjoyment of the right to health still remains a distant goal" (CESCR, 2000, para. 5). In order to alleviate this situation, the CESCR lists several "International obligations" (para. 38–42, 45). It is explicitly stated that "[s]tates parties have to respect the enjoyment of the right to health in other countries [...], wherever possible, and provide the necessary aid when required" (para. 39), and that

> For the avoidance of any doubt, the Committee wishes to emphasize that it is particularly incumbent on States parties and other actors in a position to assist, to provide 'international assistance and cooperation, especially economic and technical' which enable developing countries to fulfil their core obligations (CESCR, 2000, para. 45).

Whereas the preceding argument refers to a right to healthcare at an international level and duties of states to assist other states in fulfilling that right, Narveson lists several other arguments against a universal right to healthcare by denoting problems of universal health coverage financed by an insurance system that rests on the high insurance premiums of the rich. In his objection to a universal right to healthcare, Narveson, thus, identifies at least three problems with realising that right at the national level.

Firstly, Narveson argues from a libertarian perspective that if there was agreement on the duty of the rich to finance healthcare for the poor, there would be no need for legal enforcement of this principle, as it could be ensured that the poor's healthcare would be covered by the charitable donations of the rich: "If we think it that good, we will buy it out of our own free will" (Narveson, 2011, p. 563). This argument ignores charitability's inability to organise and justly allocate the healthcare fund collected for the poor, especially as donations are always relative to personal preferences of those who donate (Buchanan, 1984, p. 69f.).

Narveson further argues that there is not "one standard health insurance that would plainly be best for everyone" (Narveson, 2011, p. 570). Here, the author overlooks that the ICESCR does not recommend implementing a single insurance scheme in any of its member states but to alleviate possible threats to the universal right to health by private insurances (cf. CESCR, 2000, para. 35). There is no reason why there could not be more than one insurance. After all, the 'one-for-all approach' would only be a foundation that could be complemented by private insurances (cf. Pellegrino, 1994, pp. 314f.). Or there could even be a system that includes several such foundational, public, insurances, among which people can choose in alignment with their preferences regarding minimal differences in the additional benefits these insurances offer, and which are reflected in insurance premiums, as, for example, is the case in Germany.[2]

Eventually, Narveson argues that from rights, like the right to healthcare, does not follow a governmental securement of these rights (cf. Narveson, 2011, p. 567). This conflicts with the CESCR's (2000) list of "State parties' obligations" (para. 30–45). Furthermore, the rationale that there is no duty of states to pay for medical education (Narveson, 2011, p. 565) can be refuted by pointing to the ICESCR: "Higher education shall be made equally accessible to all, on the basis of capacity, by every appropriate means, and in particular by the progressive introduction of free education" (ICESCR, 1966, article 13, para. 2, c).

Along with further arguments in favour of a universal right to healthcare (e.g. Daniels, 2001; Ruger, 2006; Hessler and Buchanan, 2012; Buchanan, 1984; Buyx, 2008; Green, 2004), it can, therefore, be concluded that there is a universal right to healthcare.

2.4 Agent-neutral and agent-relative right to health(care) (cf. Nagel, 1986)

As has been concluded above, with Nagel, the objectivity of values can be presumed. I have argued that from the intrinsic value of human beings follows the objective value of health and healthcare, as both are instrumental for human

---

[2]   For a discussion of different types of healthcare and insurance systems cf. also Buch *et al.* in this volume.

beings. Nagel arrives at the objective standpoint necessary for assessing and 'discovering' (Nagel, 1986, p. 146) values by a "view from nowhere" (title of his book), i.e. from outside the world. This perspective allows for an assessment of what is objectively, i.e. reasonably, valuable for a specific person in a specific situation, or even for all persons in that situation. It differs from a subjective assessment of the situation, i.e. from how human beings, like me or you, can subjectively arrive at an answer to the question: "What is valuable for me?", as, only from an objective standpoint, according to Nagel, this question can be answered in a normatively reasonable and perhaps normatively true manner. Similar to "theoretical reasoning", where "objectivity is advanced when we form a new conception of reality that includes ourselves as components" (p. 138), "[w]e try to arrive at normative judgments, with motivational content, from an impersonal standpoint" (pp. 138f.). Therefore, we view the world from outside, where what is valuable for me is decided upon an impersonal view on myself as an answer to the question what for "that *person*" (p. 155; emphasis in original), which happens to be me, is reasonably valuable. As "that *person*" can also be another person, according to Nagel, it is possible to objectively assess what is valuable for a specific person, e.g. me and you. What we arrive at by this method are personal or agent-relative values and reasons (cf. p. 153).

It can easily be understood that the agent-relative value of health and of healthcare can be attributed to every human being, as it has been concluded above that the value of health and of healthcare is universal. Therefore, there is not only an agent-relative value of health(care), but also, to again implement Nagel's terminology, an agent-neutral, or impersonal, value (cf. p. 152) of health(care). It is much more complicated to arrive at agent-neutral values, as a fully objective perspective might abstract from any agents that could have and for whom there could be value: "It is true that with nothing to go on but a conception of the world from nowhere, one would have no way of telling whether anything had value" (p. 147). Nagel, therefore, suggests to simply consider all agents at once when trying to arrive at impersonal values, i.e. not to abstract from personal viewpoints but to collectively put them together:

> We are thinking from no particular point of view about how to regard a world which contains points of view. What exists inside those points of view can be considered from outside to have some sort of value simply as part of what is happening in the world, and the value assigned to it should be that which it overwhelmingly appears to have from the inside. (Nagel, 1986, p. 161)

Consequently, it is possible, with Nagel, to assume that there are agent-relative as well as agent-neutral values. The value of health and of healthcare is such. As it has been argued above that from these values follows a right to health and to healthcare, this right can as well be specified so that it comprises agent-relative rights of specific persons to health(care) and an agent-neutral right to health(care). Both are universal rights, as everyone has them.

In the debate on the value of healthcare, DeCamp (2019) refers to agent-relative and agent-neutral value as well. He uses the terminology slightly differently to Nagel and does not explicitly refer to him. I will refer to the divergence in the discussion section of my paper (section 4). For an overview on agent-neutral versus agent-relative reasons, one may also read Ridge (2017) and Schroeder (2016).

3   From the universal right to health(care) follows a sustainable right to health(care)

3.1   Traditional concept of sustainability (cf. WCED, 1987; Elkington, 1999; MacDonald and Norman, 2007)

In the following, it will be conceptualized how from the universal right to health and to healthcare follows a sustainable right to health and to healthcare. Before doing so, I will briefly summarise what I refer to as the economic, or the traditional, concept of sustainability, which originated in economic sciences and has been discussed in business ethics. In 1987, the UN's World Commission on Environment and Development (WCED) adopted the so-called Brundtland Report *Our Common Future*, where it set forth in paragraph 1 of the conclusion of chapter 2:

> Sustainable development is development that meets the needs of the present without compromising the ability of future generations to meet their own needs. It contains within it two key concepts: the concept of 'needs', in particular the essential needs of the world's poor, to which overriding priority should be given; and the idea of limitations imposed by the state of technology and social organization on the environment's ability to meet present and future needs. (WCED, 1987, chapter 2)

Thereafter, in the 1990s, economist John Elkington formed the concept of a "triple bottom line" sustainability approach aiming at measurability of the sustainability of businesses. Since then, the concept has quickly been widely adopted "in management, consulting, investing, and NGO circles" (Norman and MacDonald, 2004, p. 243), as well as broadly discussed from the perspective of business ethics. Whilst a literature review of the discussion on the ethical aspects of the triple bottom line approach is beyond the scope of this paper, it could start by analysing the vast amount of articles including the term "triple bottom line" that have been published in the *Journal of Business Ethics*.

Like the WCED, Elkington defines sustainability with reference to future generations: "Sustainability is the principle of ensuring that our actions today do not limit the range of economic, social, and environmental options open to future generations" (Elkington, 1999, p. 20). This has been the point of origination of my interest in his approach for a discussion of the value of health and healthcare from an ethical perspective. For if there is a universal right to health and healthcare, it follows that not only at present but also in the future, entitlements to this right uphold, i.e., as has been stated above, that to grant the right to health to everyone, a healthy environment, healthy social conditions, and the provision of healthcare do not only have to be created but also sustained. Therefore, the right to health and to healthcare if universal, needs to be sustainable and sustained for future generations. In cases where potential health services or health technologies would or could negatively affect the health of future generations, the sustainable right to health and to healthcare is violated. This is one reason why a potential health technology that generates inheritable changes in the patient is regarded as ethically unacceptable, and why the aspect of effect on future generations is an important ethical criterion in the debate on germline genome editing, as germline genome editing might be unsustainable. In search of an approach to integrate the aspect of future generations in a broader conception of the value of healthcare, the concept of sustainability, therefore, presented itself as highly suitable.

However, Elkington's triple bottom line approach cannot be copied, as it stands, for a concept of sustainable health and healthcare, especially since his aim is to use the approach for business accounting. He, thus, takes an economic perspective that is not suitable for an ethical view on the right to health(care). By including the "social bottom line", the "economic bottom line", and the "environmental bottom line" into his approach (pp. 73f.), he argues that all of these can be taken together to "assess a company's [...] performance", in the way that "accountants pull together, record and analyze a wide range of numerical data" (p. 74). The hierarchy of the three bottom lines be defined by their interdependencies: "Society depends on the economy – and the economy depends on the global ecosystem, whose health represents the ultimate bottom line" (p. 73). Because Elkington especially points to values that influenced his approach (in a chapter of his book from 1999 named accordingly, pp. 123–158), "such as concern for future generations" (p. 124), it is justified to see his intention in the fact that the social and the environmental bottom line are supposed to integrate ethical aspects into business accounting. Therefore, it would have been necessary that he clarified why he, on the one hand, separates the economic bottom line from the other two, ethically oriented, bottom lines but, on the other hand, frames the entire approach as one of accounting, hence, one of economics, and not one of ethics. As MacDonald and Norman (2007) have argued in response to Pava (2007) (Pava (2007) responded to the paper by Norman and MacDonald (2004) quoted above):

> the accounting paradigm is inappropriate as a comprehensive methodology for the ethical evaluation of a firm and its operations. Crucially *qualitative* distinctions – especially deontic distinctions between different kinds of obligations and responsi-

bilities – would be bulldozed over by an entirely *quantitative* evaluation scheme. (MacDonald and Norman, 2007, p. 112; emphasis in original)

Aligning with John Elkington (1999) but considering the criticism of his approach and in recourse to the WCED's definition of sustainable development, I understand the traditional concept of sustainability as including social aspects (as a concern for present as well as future generations), economic aspects (as the "[s]ociety depends on the economy"; Elkington, 1999, p. 73), and environmental aspects (as "the economy depends on the global ecosystem"; ibid.; but especially as society depends on the health of the environment).

3.2 The concept of a sustainable right to health

Daniel D. Reidpath and colleagues, in their article "Is the right to health compatible with sustainability?" (*Journal of Global Health*, 2015) argue that the universal right to health as understood by the ICESCR (1966) conflicts with sustainability (Reidpath *et al.*, 2015, p. 1). Measuring sustainability by reference to a country's per capita ecological footprint, and assessing realisation of the right to the highest attainable standard of health (HASH) by taking life expectancy as a HASH point, an analysis of 147 countries, conducted in 2008, revealed that countries with the highest HASH point were significantly less sustainable than countries with lower HASH points (p. 2). The authors, therefore, claim to replace the right to the highest attainable standard of health by "a fundamental human right to the highest *sustainable* standard of health" (p. 3; emphasis in original).

As has been shown in the previous section, I do not agree with Reidpath and colleagues' negative answer to the question "Is the right to health compatible with sustainability?". I understand the universal right to health as comprising a sustainable right to health, as the latter follows from the former. I, therefore, do agree with the request of Reidpath and colleagues to alleviate the problem that "at a population level, the highest attainable standard of health is a standard that is achieved (or progressively realised) through unsustainable levels of consumption" (Reidpath *et al.*, 2015, p. 1). In order to mitigate this problem, I suggest that the universal right to health can, firstly, only be realised at an international level, which transcends the "population level", and, secondly, must be understood as a sustainable right to health that includes the right to health of future generations.

However, I do not think that such a concept of a sustainable right to health is limited to the mitigation of "unsustainable levels of consumption", but that it is also suitable to prevent problems resulting from the implementation of certain health technologies or specific practices in healthcare, inasmuch as these technologies or practices might result in a successful treatment of one patient at the cost of the health or even the life of another human being. Here again, I may refer to the example of assisted reproductive medicine.

As in germline genome editing, the embryo that is edited might be successfully treated but might, nevertheless, bequeath unintended effects of the treatment to its descendants and, accordingly, pass on a negative effect to the health of future generations (e.g., cf. Petre, 2017; Schöne-Seifert, 2017), so too, in another form of reproductive medicine, negative effects on the health of human beings are negative side effects. Selective embryo transfer following in vitro fertilization or preimplantation genetic diagnosis is an apt example. These health technologies are applied to cure the infertility of couples, hence, in respect for the agent-relative reproductive rights (as part of the universal right to health) of patients who are unable to have (healthy) children naturally. Respect for these agent-relative rights may disregard the agent-neutral right to health (and life) of the embryos that are discarded or selected against in the process of the treatment, at least if these embryos have intrinsic value that justifies their agent-neutral right to health (including a right to life). In both examples, granting of the right to health disregards the sustainable right to health of future generations.

If it is considered that, also in the process of germline genome editing, embryo selection cannot be avoided (e.g., cf. Ranisch, 2020, p. 64; Wells, 2019, p. 347), those embryos that are successfully edited are those whose right to health is respected, but it is respected at the cost of the discarding of other embryos in the process of the application of the technology. Hence, respect for the right to health of successfully edited embryos in the case of genome editing comes at the cost of disregard for the right to health (and life) of other embryos that have been created at around the same time as the successfully edited embryos, and are, therefore, (from the point of view of the successfully edited embryos) not members of future generations but of the same generation. Similarly, one can argue that the right to health of members of the same generation is affected by healthcare for other members of that same generation in cases of "[t]he prevention, treatment and control of epidemic, endemic, occupational and other diseases" (ICESCR, 1966, Art. 12, para. 2, c), such as immunization, but also as triage and allocation of scarce resources (e.g., cf. ÖGARI, 2020). The latter has been the focus of medical ethics during the SARS-CoV-2/COVID-19 pandemic that, at the time of writing this article, remains an unsolved global problem.

Summing up these examples, it can be stated that viewing the right to health from the perspective of sustainability does allow for an approach to realise the agent-neutral right to health, including the right to health of future generations as well as of all members of the global community of present generations. Thus, one aspect of the concept of a sustainable right to health resembles the component "societal aspects" of the traditional concept of sustainability. Furthermore, it is especially important to sustain healthy social conditions to fulfil the right to health inasmuch as it transcends the right to healthcare (cf. CESCR, 2000, para. 4).

As has also been shown in the examples, the agent-relative right to health of specific individuals in specific situations is another important aspect of a sustainable right to health. To only reiterate one example, the reproductive health is important when deciding whether to undertake preimplantation genetic diagnosis. Equally important in this case may be the right to health and life of specific embryos that might be discarded in the process of the infertility treatment. Depending on the point of view, either of those rights can be described as agent-relative, as either of those rights indeed is agent-relative as well as agent-neutral. However, when the perspective of the (potential) parents is taken, their reproductive rights are agent-relative as they result from their specific intrinsic value as human beings.

Especially when conceptualizing the sustainable right to healthcare (see next section), the patient in a specific patient-physician relationship can be viewed as the agent whose agent-relative right to healthcare needs to be primarily considered (cf. DeCamp, 2019), although it may be possible to discuss with the patient how treatment for her/him influences the availability of treatment for other patients through economic aspects, i.e. costs of her/his individual treatment (cf. DeCamp 2019, pp. 238f.; Pearson, 2000). A third aspect of a sustainable right to health, therefore, is the economic aspect. Contrary to Elkington's approach on sustainability, from an ethical perspective, the economic aspect can only be viewed as instrumental to the fulfilment of the agent-relative and agent-neutral sustainable right to health. Nevertheless, this aspect resembles the economic aspect of the traditional concept of sustainability.

Finally, a fourth aspect is similar to the traditional concept of sustainability; this is the inclusion of environmental aspects into a sustainable right to health, as it is especially important to sustain not only healthy social but also healthy environmental conditions in order to fulfil the right to health inasmuch as it transcends the right to healthcare (cf. CESCR, 2000, para. 4).

It can, thus, be concluded that the concept of a sustainable right to health comprises the agent-relative right to health (health of individual with intrinsic value, in a specific situation), the agent-neutral right to health (health of each individual within the global society, at present and in future; healthy social conditions to sustain the right to health), economic aspects (inasmuch as they are necessary to fulfil agent-relative and agent-neutral rights to health), environmental aspects (healthy environmental conditions to sustain the right to health).

3.3 The concept of a sustainable right to healthcare

As there is a universal and sustainable right to health, there is also a universal and sustainable right to healthcare for, as stated in ICESCR (1966) and CESCR (2000), the right to health encompasses the right to healthcare. This has been outlined above. Furthermore, in the previous section, the four components of a sustainable right to health have been described. Those already comprise the three components of the sustainable right to healthcare.

The sustainable right to healthcare, thus, encompasses the agent-relative right to healthcare (of an individual patient, such as in a specific patient-physician relationship; cf. DeCamp, 2019, pp. 235ff.), the agent-neutral right to healthcare (of each present and future member of society), economic aspects (especially of the health economy; no economic interests that are beyond moral interests, i.e. none that exceed guaranteeing a sustainable right to healthcare).

Because the sustainable right to healthcare depicts the component of the sustainable right to health that refers to healthcare, it does not include the other components and conditions for health. As such, its scope is narrower. This is the reason why environmental aspects are not included as a fourth component.

4 Discussion of the economic aspects of the right to healthcare in consideration of a possible conflict between agent-relative and agent-neutral rights

4.1 Selected aspects of the debate on healthcare rationing in different countries

With the preceding two paragraphs, the argument outlined at the beginning of this paper that has been discussed in sections 2 and 3 concluded with an ethical conceptualization of a sustainable right to health and a sustainable right to healthcare. As depicted in the section on the traditional concept of sustainability, one of the main motivations for the development of this approach has been the urge to conceptualize the value of healthcare and the right to health in a way that integrates future generations' rights. Another driving point was to find a way, at least on a broad, conceptual level, to integrate economic aspects of the value of healthcare into an ethical approach on the right to health.[3]

---

[3]   For the economic aspects of the value of healthcare see the contributions of Buch et al., and of Ubels to this volume. Further discussions of ethical aspects of the value of

This issue is especially pressing considering that economic decisions can have a considerable impact on the stability of the health system. That might result in threats to the long-term availability of healthcare, for example, if physicians' values regarding care for their patients conflict with health reforms that aim at saving costs. This was the case in New Zealand, where many young physicians left the country to practice in Australia instead, where economic pressures were less acute (cf. Brunton, 2017).

As several contributions in this volume on the value of healthcare can be found that relate to healthcare in various countries,[4] it might be suitable to refer to further examples of country-specific discussions on economic aspects of healthcare, but not without clarifying that those are eventually relevant for other countries where similar problems may arise or are already prevalent (cf. Brunton, 2017, p. 720).

Chaar and Lee (2012) might be mentioned; they discuss the impact of direct-to-consumer advertising of drugs by pharmaceutical companies on costs in the Australian public healthcare system.

For the United Kingdom, the Centre for Evidence-Based Medicine's (CEBM) 2019 report *Defining Value-based Healthcare in the NHS* might be quoted. It also refers to the National Institute for Health and Care Excellence's (NICE) "systems of resource allocation" (CEBM, 2019, p. 7). The report defines: "Value-based healthcare is the equitable, sustainable and transparent use of the available resources to achieve better outcomes and experiences for every person" (CEBM, 2019, p. 3), and considers the environmental as well as economically sustainable use of health(care) resources (e.g., cf. p. 8). The CEBM's understanding of value-based healthcare might, therefore, be similar to the conceptualization I present in this paper.

In Germany, the German Interdisciplinary Association for Intensive and Emergency Medicine (Deutsche Interdisziplinäre Vereinigung für Intensiv- und Notfallmedizin, DIVI) restricts economic considerations in evaluations of the reasonableness of intensive care medicine, on the one hand, to those that have been socio-politically justified. On the other hand, the DIVI acknowledges deviations from the economic efficiency dictate in case-by-case-decisions (cf. DIVI, 2016, section 1). This, as well, might resonate with my approach. Furthermore, the German Society for Internal Medicine (Deutsche Gesellschaft für Innere Medizin, DGIM) adopted a *Clinic Codex: Medicine before economics* in 2017 (Schumm-Draeger *et al.*, 2017), which is consistent with the limitations of the economic aspects of a sustainable right to health(care) described above.

---

healthcare can be found in the contributions by Stutzin Donoso, Napiwodzka and Parsons.

4   Steigenberger *et al.* refer to health technology assessment (HTA) in Germany; Napiwodzka specifically takes the perspective of the Polish healthcare system.

4.2 Inability to pay as a possible restriction to the right to healthcare?

In the past, the debate on economic restrictions to the universal right to healthcare has considered whether the inability to pay could be a valid reason for physicians to step out of their contract with the patient, i.e. to disregard agent-relative rights to healthcare of those who are unable to pay, in order to save their resources for the rest of society and their agent-neutral rights (cf. Mehlman and Massey, 1994). These considerations may also be restricted to those who voluntarily risk their own health, e.g. through dangerous sports (cf. Veatch, 1980), or to those who voluntarily decided to pay for only minimal insurance coverage in a system of economic competition between health insurers and are then unable to pay for their healthcare by themselves in cases that are not covered by their minimal insurance (cf. Menzel, 1987).

As Pellegrino argues in response to Mehlman and Massey (1994), and as I have referred to above in response to one of Narveson's (2011) arguments (see section 2), because of "the ethical obligations of physicians that are inherent in the physician-patient relationship" (Pellegrino, 1994, p. 309), inability to pay is an invalid argument to withhold care from "the poor" (p. 313), or practically from anyone, as every human being has a right to healthcare.

4.3 Disregard for agent-relative rights to healthcare in Porter's economic definition of the value of healthcare (cf. DeCamp, 2019; Porter, 2010)

DeCamp, inspired by Pellegrino, identifies the latter aspect as agent-relative. He argues that an economic definition of, or, as he calls it, the contemporary view of the value of healthcare is entirely agent-neutral, whereas an ethical definition be "*agent-relative* (relative to the patient)" (DeCamp, 2019, p. 235; emphasis in original). Slightly different from Nagel's understanding of the term, DeCamp refers to agent-neutrality as an economically calculating approach that assigns greater value to what has the same or an equally 'large' health outcome but costs less. He, thereby, refers to how Michael Porter defines the value of healthcare: "value defined as the health outcomes achieved per dollar spent" (Porter, 2010, p. 2477); "value is defined as outcomes relative to cost" (ibid.). This does not resemble how I have defined agent-neutral value and rights (see corresponding section in section 2).

I, nevertheless, agree with DeCamp in that, firstly, (a) economic aspects of a discussion on the value of and rights to health(care) are foremost necessary to secure sustainable agent-neutral rights to health(care), and that, secondly,

(b) as has already been outlined above (see section on the concept of a sustainable right to health in section 3), agent-relative rights conflict with these agent-neutral rights.

Regarding the first aspect (a) Porter's account on the value of healthcare clearly needs to be rejected. Insofar as value, in Porter's definition, is dependent on a relation of health outcome and healthcare spending, it is not defined independently of economic considerations because the value of healthcare ultimately depends on healthcare spending if a slightly different – and slightly better – health outcome is achieved by a very different amount of "dollar[s] spent", i.e. if by spending $ 1 Million for healthcare A, a slightly better health outcome can be achieved than by spending $ 5,000 for healthcare B. Despite the better health outcome of healthcare A, according to Michael Porter's definition, the value of healthcare B will be higher than the value of healthcare A. It is, therefore, evident that Porter's definition is almost exclusively economic. It is, however, problematic that Porter does not define what he means by "health outcome".

Regarding the second of these two aspects (b), I want to once again clarify that the right to health and to healthcare is an agent-neutral right because everyone has this right, in Nagel's words: to act in such a way to promote anybody's health, regardless whose health it is, has an objective reason. Respecting the intrinsic value of each individual is priority number one. Therefore, it seems reasonable to argue that any decision that not merely indirectly but directly disregards the intrinsic value of any present or future individual cannot be justified. Only when there is no such disregard, the agent-neutral right of society (at present and in future) requires the inclusion of economic discussions and the search for a healthcare system (and health economy) that is universally accessible and can be sustained for as long as possible (cf. Reidpath *et al.*, 2015).

5   Limitations and implications

Whether there are (objective) values at all has not been conclusively proven; the debate on Nagel's attempt at proving this has also not been analysed, at any rate in this paper, as the present article is more application-oriented. Further theoretical work, therefore, needs to be done to investigate whether there actually is such a thing as an (objective) sustainable right to health and to healthcare.

Even if there is such a right, another issue remains controversial. The problem that agent-relative and agent-neutral rights to health(care) may conflict, which is reflected by economic discussions on how to ration healthcare in a just way, has not been definitively untangled in this paper. The attempt (especially at the very end of section 4) to solve it by referring to intrinsic value is, firstly, only superficial, as possible counterarguments have not been analysed and refuted. Secondly, this attempt lacks consideration of literature relevant to the concept of intrinsic values but, instead, only ties up with Nagel's introduction of this type of value.

A possible implication of the ethical conceptualization of a sustainable right to health(care) may be to include within HTA, where it is recommended by literature that ethical aspects become more dominant (e.g., cf. Hofmann, 2005; INAHTA, 2005; WHO, 2015), a section that considers whether the health technology assessed conflicts with a sustainable right to health(care) not only of present but also of future members of the entire, global society.[5] Details of this right and, accordingly, of the aspects that could be evaluated in such a rubric of an HTA still need to be developed (especially as I am not an expert on HTA, this approach is only a suggestion from the perspective of ethics). Here, connections between HTA and technology impact assessment (in German: *Technikfolgenabschätzung*) need to be specified.

Finally, there are several health technologies that can be evaluated more comprehensively if discussed from a sustainability perspective. Apart from those that have been mentioned throughout the paper (e.g. immunization and other forms of "control of epidemic [...] and other diseases", ICESCR, 1966, Art. 12, para. 2, c; assisted reproductive technologies, such as preimplantation genetic diagnosis and germline genome editing), those include antibiotics and the discussion of antimicrobial resistance of future patients. These examples would benefit from an analysis with reference to the concept of a sustainable right to health(care) proposed here for the first time. However, I acknowledge that this concept is still very much open to amendments and specifications.

Acknowledgments: The work has been supported by the German Research Foundation (DFG), grant number: 409799774 as part of the ethical subproject of the DFG-funded project "Comparative Assessment of Genome and Epigenome Editing in Medicine – Ethical, Legal and Social Implications" (COMPASS-ELSI), which is conducted by Prof. Dr. med. Dr. phil. Eva C. Winkler. I would like to thank the organisers and the other participants of the international conference for young scholars "Defining the value of medical interventions – Normative and empirical challenges" (Fuerth/Nuremberg, September 16–20, 2019), in particular Francisca Stutzin Donoso and Jordan Parsons. I also thank Michael Parker, Christoph Schickhardt, Anja Köngeter, Martin Jungkunz, and especially Eva Winkler for their valuable comments on the ideas presented in this paper.

---

[5]   Cf. Steigenberger *et al.*'s contribution to this volume for a discussion of HTA.

References

Baumrin, S. B. (2012), "Why There Is No Right to Health Care", in Rhodes, R., Battin, M., and Silvers, A. (Eds.) *Medicine and Social Justice: Essays on the Distribution of Health Care,* 2nd edition, Oxford University Press, New York, pp. 91–96.

Brunton, M. (2017), "Risking the Sustainability of the Public Health System: Ethical Conundrums and Ideologically Embedded Reform", *Journal of Business Ethics,* Vol. 142 No. 4, pp. 719–734.

Buchanan, A. E. (1984), "The Right to a Decent Minimum of Health Care", *Philosophy & Public Affairs,* Vol. 13 No. 1, pp. 55–78.

Buyx, A. M. (2008), "Personal responsibility for health as a rationing criterion: why we don't like it and why maybe we should", *Journal of Medical Ethics,* Vol. 34 No. 12, pp. 871–874.

CEBM: Centre for Evidence-Based Medicine at the University of Oxford (2019), "Defining Value-based Healthcare in the NHS: Report 2019/04", Available at: https://www.cebm.net/2019/04/defining-value-based-healthcare-in-the-nhs/ (accessed 2 December 2020).

Chaar, B. B., and Lee, J. (2012), "Role of Socioeconomic Status on Consumers' Attitudes Towards DTCA of Prescription Medicine in Australia", *Journal of Business Ethics,* Vol. 105 No. 4, pp. 447–460.

CESCR: Committee on Economic, Social and Cultural Rights (2000), "General Comment No. 14: The Right to the Highest Attainable Standard of Health (Art. 12), adopted at the Twenty-second Session of the Committee on Economic, Social and Cultural Rights, on 11 August 2000 (Contained in Document E/C.12/2000/4)", United Nations, Available at: https://www.refworld.org/pdfid/4538838d0.pdf (accessed 2 December 2020).

Cummiskey, D. (2004), "The right to die and the right to health care", in Boylan, M. (Ed.) *Public Health Policy and Ethics,* Springer Netherlands, Dordrecht, pp. 187–202.

Daniels, N. (2001), "Is There a Right to Health Care and, If So, What Does It Encompass?", in Kuhse, H., and Singer, P. (Eds.) *A Companion to Bioethics,* 2nd edition, Wiley-Blackwell, Oxford, pp. 362–372.

DeCamp, M. (2019), "Toward a Pellegrino-inspired theory of value in health care", *Theoretical Medicine and Bioethics,* Vol. 40 No. 3, pp. 231–241.

DIVI: Deutsche Interdisziplinäre Vereinigung für Intensiv- und Notfallmedizin, Sektion Ethik (2016), "Grenzen der Sinnhaftigkeit von Intensivmedizin: Positionspapier", Available at: https://www.divi.de/empfehlungen/publikationen/grenzen-der-sinnhaftigkeit-von-intensivmedizin/viewdocument/67 (accessed 2 December 2020).

Elkington, J. (1999), Cannibals with forks: the triple bottom line of 21st century business, Capstone, Oxford.

Green, M. (2004), "Global Justice and Health: Is Health Care a Basic Right", in Boylan, M. (Ed.) *Public Health Policy and Ethics,* Springer Netherlands, Dordrecht, pp. 203–221.

Hessler, K., and Buchanan, A. (2012), "Equality, Democracy, and the Human Right to Health Care", in Rhodes, R., Battin, M., and Silvers, A. (Eds.) *Medicine and Social Justice: Essays on the Distribution of Health Care,* 2nd edition, New York, Oxford University Press pp. 97–104.

Hofmann, B. (2005), "On value-judgements and ethics in health technology assessment", *Poiesis & Praxis,* Vol. 3 No. 4, pp. 277–295.

ICESCR: International Covenant on Economic, Social and Cultural Rights (1966), "Resolution 2200A (XXI) of 16 December 1966, entry into force 3 January 1976, in accordance with article 27", United Nations, Available at: https://www.ohchr.org/en/professionalinterest/pages/cescr.aspx (accessed 2 December 2020.

INAHTA: International Network of Agencies for HTA Ethics Working Group (2005), "Working Group on Handling Ethical Issues: Final report, June 2005", Available at: https://www.inahta.org/wp-content/uploads/2014/03/Final-report-Ethics-in-HTA-Nov-07.pdf (accessed 2 December 2020).

MacDonald, C., and Norman, W. (2007), "Rescuing the Baby from the Triple-Bottom-Line Bathwater: A Reply to Pava", *Business Ethics Quarterly,* Vol. 17 No. 1, pp. 111–114.

Mehlman, M. J., and Massey, S. R. (1994), "The Patient-Physician Relationship and the Allocation of Scarce Resources: A Law and Economics Approach", *Kennedy Institute of Ethics Journal,* Vol. 4 No. 4, pp. 291–308.

Menzel, P. T. (1987), "Economic Competition in Health Care: A Moral Assessment", *The Journal of Medicine and Philosophy,* Vol. 12 No. 1, pp. 63–84.

Nagel, T. (1986), *The view from nowhere,* Oxford University Press, Oxford, New York.

Narveson, J. (2011), "The Medical Minimum: Zero", *Journal of Medicine and Philosophy,* Vol. 36 No. 6, pp. 558–571.

Norman, W., and MacDonald, C. (2004), "Getting to the Bottom of 'Triple Bottom Line'", *Business Ethics Quarterly,* Vol. 14 No. 2, pp. 243–262.

ÖGARI: Österreichische Gesellschaft für Anästhesiologie, Reanimation und Intensivmedizin (2020), "Allokation intensivmedizinischer Ressourcen aus Anlass der Covid-19-Pandemie: Klinisch-ethische Empfehlungen für Beginn, Durchführung und Beendigung von Intensivtherapie bei Covid-19-PatientInnen, Statement der Arbeitsgruppe Ethik der Österreichischen Gesellschaft für Anästhesiologie, Reanimation und Intensivmedizin (ARGE Ethik ÖGARI) vom 17.03.2020", Available at: https://www.oegari.at/web_files/cms_daten/covid-19_ressourcenallokation_gari-statement_v1.7_final_2020-03-17.pdf (accessed 2 December 2020).

Pava, M. L. (2007), "A Response to 'Getting to the Bottom of 'Triple Bottom Line''", *Business Ethics Quarterly,* Vol. 17 No. 1, pp. 105–110.

Pearson, S. D. (2000), "Caring and Cost: The Challenge for Physician Advocacy", *Annals of Internal Medicine,* Vol. 133 No. 2, pp. 148–153.

Pellegrino, E. (1994), "Allocation of Resources at the Bedside: The Intersections of Economics, Law and Ethics", *Kennedy Institute of Ethics Journal,* Vol. 4 No. 4, pp. 309–317.

Petre, I. (2017), "Future Generations and the Justifiability of Germline Engineering", *The Journal of Medicine and Philosophy,* Vol. 42 No. 3, pp. 328–341.

Porter, M. E. (2010), "What Is Value in Health Care?", *The New England Journal of Medicine,* Vol. 363 No. 26, pp. 2477–2481.

Ranisch, R. (2020), "Germline genome editing versus preimplantation genetic diagnosis: Is there a case in favour of germline interventions?", *Bioethics,* Vol. 34 No. 1, pp. 60–69.

Reidpath, D. D., Gruskin, S., and Allotey, P. (2015), "Is the right to health compatible with sustainability?", *Journal of Global Health,* Vol. 5, 010301 No. 1, pp. 1–4.

Ridge, M. (2017), "Reasons for Action: Agent-Neutral vs. Agent-Relatice", in Zalta, E. N. (Ed.) *The Stanford Encyclopedia of Philosophy, Fall 2017 Edition,* Available at: https://plato.stanford.edu/archives/fall2017/entries/reasons-agent/ (accessed 2 December 2020).

Ruger, J. P. (2006), "Toward a Theory of a Right to Health: Capability and Incompletely Theorized Agreements", *Yale Journal of Law and the Humanities,* Vol. 18 No. 2, p. 3.

Schöne-Seifert, B. (2017), "Genscheren-Forschung an der menschlichen Keimbahn: Plädoyer für eine neue Debatte auch in Deutschland", *Ethik in der Medizin,* Vol. 29 No. 3, pp. 93–96.

Schroeder, M. (2016), "Value Theory", in Zalta, E. N. (Ed.) *The Stanford Encyclopedia of Philosophy, Fall 2016 Edition,* Available at: https://plato.stanford.edu/archives/fall2016/entries/value-theory/ (accessed 2 December 2020).

Schumm-Draeger, P.-M., Kapitza, T., Mann, K., Fölsch, U., and Müller-Wieland, D. (2017), "Ökonomisierung in der Medizin: Rückhalt für ärztliches Handeln", *Deutsches Ärzteblatt,* Vol. 114 No. 49, pp. 2338–2340.

Veatch, R. M. (1980), "Voluntary Riks to Health: The Ethical Issues", *The Journal of the American Medical Association,* Vol. 243 No. 1, pp. 50–55.

Wells, D., Vermeesch, J. R., and Simpson, J. L. (2019), "Current Controversies in Prenatal Diagnosis 3: Gene editing should replace embryo selection following PGD", *Prenatal Diagnosis,* Vol. 39 No. 5, pp. 344–350.

WCED: World Commission on Environment and Development (1987), "Report of the World Commission on Environment and Development: Our Common Future", United Nations, Available at: https://sustainabledevelopment.un.org/content/documents/5987our-com mon-future.pdf (accessed 2 December 2020).

WHO: World Health Organization (2015), "2015 Global Survey on Health Technology Assessment by National Authorities: Main Findings", Available at: https://www.who.int/ health-technology-assessment/MD_HTA_oct2015_final_web2.pdf (accessed 2 December 2020).

Value(s) in healthcare.
Interdisciplinary analyses

The cost-effectiveness of what in health and care?

Paul Mark Mitchell

Abstract

Assessing the value for money offered by new health technologies is playing an increasingly important role in aiding decision-making in health and care. Even in a pre-COVID-19 world, international healthcare systems were struggling to meet the demands of their patient populations and the rising cost of new health technologies, such as pharmaceuticals. With the impact of the coronavirus pandemic on the global economy and the provision of other health and care services more generally, difficult decisions will continue to be required over what basket of health and care services are available to the general population.

Health economists have developed methods to aid decision-makers who want to improve population health as the primary goal. Tools such as quality-adjusted life years (QALYs) combine health-related quality of life and quantity of life into a single outcome. QALYs allow for population health to be maximised. However, there is debate over whether the quality of life content captured by QALYs is too narrow. In addition, the aim of maximisation in health may be at odds with other goals of health and care, such as reducing health inequalities.

This chapter discusses some of the key steps involved in the construction of the QALY to value patient benefits from health and care interventions, and also how the QALY is commonly used in economic evaluation to aid healthcare decision-making. A critique and an alternative to QALYs is also provided.

Evaluating peoples capabilities has been proposed as an alternative to health focused outcomes, such as QALYs, to inform health and care decision-making. Developed initially by nobel prize winning economist and philosopher, Amartya Sen, capabilities represent what a person is able to do and be in life that they have reason to value. Although health functionings are an important component of Sen's Capability Approach, using QALYs does not fully extend the evaluative focus on to how such health outcomes and other non-health functionings are reflective of what people can and cannot do in their life that they have reason to value. Aiming to get people to a decent or sufficient level of capability also provides an alternative to the health maximisation objective commonly pursued in health economic evaluations.

Adopting a different quality of life measurement approach in health economic evaluations, as well as a new objective, has important implications for what patients and treatments are prioritised in health and care. Previous research has shown how interventions that improve quality of life for patients with mental health conditions and more severe health conditions will be more favourably treated using a capability measure. It is also recognised that health inequality has largely been neglected in the singular focus of QALY maximisation. Shifting to a "sufficient capability" objective may help address efficiency and equity concerns without the need for more complex economic evaluation frameworks that require dual objectives to deal with population health and health inequality simultaneously.

Keywords: health economics, QALY, capability approach

1 Introduction

Health economics are two words that some may be surprised to see side by side. Commonly misinterpreted as a subject that is solely focused on the economy or the wealth of nations, the subject of economics is interested in the study of choices people make and how these choices impact on different markets, including the market for health and care (Bishai and Rochaix, 2020). For a variety of reasons, the market for healthcare is very different than other markets, with a requirement of government intervention to deal with "market failures" that would otherwise occur (Morris *et al.*, 2007, pp. 125–145).

Increasingly, adopting an economic approach is undertaken in the assessment of new health technologies. Healthcare agencies who emphasise evidence-based medicine are not only interested in clinical and ethical concerns such as the quality, safety and efficacy of new health technologies, but also the cost-effectiveness of such interventions too (Taylor *et al.*, 2004).

The requirement of at least some consideration of the cost-effectiveness or value for money offered by new health technologies is also linked to another fundamental principle in health economics: the notion of scarcity. In health and care, scarcity translates to the availability of health and care where demand for healthcare exceeds supply. Health and care resources, as in the availability of health and care professionals, buildings, equipment, and medicines, are not in infinite supply in any healthcare system, however funded. Therefore, funding for additional health and care interventions means choices are required to allocate health and care resources (Morris *et al.*, 2007, p. 3).

Cost-effectiveness analysis (CEA) has become a key component in the valuation of new health technologies. CEA aims to aid decision-making by determining whether a new technology is *worth* the (typically) additional cost to the health and care system under consideration (Drummond *et al.*, 2015). The provision of a new health technology will be at the expense of existing or other new health and care resources that will not be able to be funded as a result. CEA has become synonymous with health technology assessment (Wisløff *et al.*, 2014), but it can be applied across other areas of health and care too (Hauck *et al.*, 2019).

This chapter provides an overview of some of the key ideas in the valuation of healthcare that have emerged from the sub-discipline of health economics over the past fifty years. What health economists refer to as "cost-effectiveness" in healthcare and how this is determined will receive close attention. How health economists define what is a cost-effective use of healthcare resources is not without challenge from a number of standpoints.

From a normative economics perspective (Robeyns 2017, p. 28), there are those who argue that how cost-effectiveness is typically defined by health economists is too narrow a focus on predominantly physical health outcomes and not on the broader wellbeing benefits individuals may obtain from treatment (Brazier and Tsuchiya, 2015; Coast *et al.*, 2008b). A number of researchers have made the argument for adopting the assessment of people's capabilities instead, drawing from the work of nobel prize winning economist Amartya Sen and the Capability Approach (Sen, 1993). Sen's critique of welfare economics has been used to justify a move away from the traditional rationale for assessing the costs and benefits of policies in monetary terms (Brouwer *et al.*, 2008; Coast *et al.*, 2008c). Yet, there is debate about how much of Sen's capability approach can be applied in economic evaluation to inform health and care decision-making (Coast *et al.* 2008b; Cookson, 2005).

This chapter provides an overview of the rationale for using economic evaluations to inform policy decisions more generally, before moving on to focus on how methods for economic evaluation have been uniquely shaped for application in health and care. The key steps involved in constructing patient *benefits* using the quality adjusted life year (QALY) will be detailed. Finally, an alternative economic evaluation framework based on the Capability Approach is provided for consideration as a different way economic analysis can be used to inform health and care decision-making.

2 Economic evaluation in health and care: the rationale

Economists have played an important role in influencing policy decisions. They have developed toolkits to help address questions on how a government or organisation should proceed when faced with multiple alternative courses of action. Economic evaluation is one of these toolkits used for aiding decision-making. Economic evaluation has been defined as *"the comparative analysis of alternative courses of action in terms of both their costs and consequences"* (Drummond *et al.*, 2015, p. 4).

The most straightforward and commonly used economic evaluation outside of health and care is called cost-benefit analysis (CBA). Essentially, in CBA if the monetary benefits outweigh the costs of introducing a new policy, the new policy is net beneficial and should proceed, and vice-versa (Drummond *et al.*, 2015, p. 10). The origins of CBA have been dated back as far as the 1840s, when French civil engineer turned economist, Jules Dupuit, wanted to determine the optimum strategy for introducing a toll on a new bridge (Ekelund, 1968). More recently, CBA ranges from providing evidence to help decide whether to build a high speed rail line from the north of England to London (DfT, 2020a), to more local decisions, such as whether a core UK city should build a large indoor arena to regenerate a derelict city centre site (KPMG, 2018).

Key to all CBA are that the costs and benefits of a policy are measured in the same unit (i.e. in monetary terms), making it relatively straightforward to compare cost and benefits to one another and decide if a policy represents value for money. Typically, the costs and benefits focus on economic impacts, in terms of the monetary cost of a policy compared to the monetary benefits, such as predicted Gross Domestic Product (GDP) growth following increased productivity; for example, the economic growth opportunities offered by the building of a new airport terminal (DfT, 2017). The aim of CBA is to maximise the benefits to society in monetary terms, with the welfare economic rationale of adopting a utilitarian maximisation objective as the social welfare function. This objective argues that society will be better off so long as the average population utility levels, in terms of individuals happiness or fulfilling preference satisfaction – commonly proxied by income – are increasing (Brouwer *et al.*, 2008).[1]

The sub-discipline of health economics has developed rapidly in just over sixty years. Kenneth Arrow was an influential figure in the foundation of health economics. Arrow recognised that the healthcare market required greater public intervention than other markets in society due to market failure in healthcare related to uncertainty in the treatment and need for medical intervention (Arrow, 1963). The argument has been made that typical CBA evaluations are not appropriate in healthcare, as it would involve challenging ethical questions for practical use, such as putting a direct monetary value on life, as well as issues of income influencing the willingness to pay estimates of individuals – thereby use of CBA could favour interventions for those with larger incomes (Coast, 2004). CBA is rarely applied in practice in health and

---

[1]   See chapter by Ubels in this publication for further details on utilitarianism in economics.

care, yet some notable attempts in using it have been made (McIntosh *et al.*, 2010).

Health economics represents a broad array of research that aims to answer specific economic questions related to health and care (Jones, 2020). A large component of health economics research has been involved in the development of alternative economic evaluation methods aimed specifically at healthcare and addressing some of the issues with using CBA in healthcare. Health economic evaluations have become particularly prominent in healthcare decision-making for new health technologies, as national regulatory bodies such as the National Institute for Health and Care Excellence (NICE) in England and similar bodies internationally require economic evaluations to be conducted before new health technologies are adopted by the national healthcare system (Rowen *et al.*, 2017). Although such methods are not routinely applied equally in all high-income countries, with Germany (Caro *et al.*, 2010) and the United States (Garrison *et al.*, 2018) notable exceptions, their increasing use internationally suggests a need for evidence to help in controlling the costs of health and care in a way that meets the requirement of both healthcare consumers (i.e. patients) and their providers.

It has already been discussed that the aim in standard welfare economic analysis is to maximise individuals utility, but it has been argued that such an approach is inappropriate when it comes to healthcare – how happy a person is may not be the only consideration we want to account for in healthcare decision-making (Sen, 2002). Instead, health economists have developed methods than aim to maximise patient health gains from health and care interventions.

Two areas in particular are given prominence in CEA (also referred to as *cost-utility analysis* by health economists (Drummond *et al.*, 2015, p. 11)). Health gains are measured in terms of gains in life years from interventions, an important objective for some healthcare interventions. In addition, the health-related quality of life (Karimi and Brazier, 2016) changes from an intervention may also be important if the intervention is not only aimed at life extension. Even for life extending interventions, it is also helpful to know the quality of life experienced in that life extended period. Therefore, CEA moves away from a common currency across costs and benefits in an attempt to account for dual considerations of improved health-related quality of life and quantity of life.

3 Health economic evaluation: key steps

3.1 Defining evaluation perspective

An important aspect in any economic evaluation is to consider what is known as *the perspective* that is appropriate for the decision-making context at hand. Health economic evaluations in some jurisdictions, such as in England, take a healthcare perspective as the reference case economic evaluation in the assessment of new health technologies (NICE, 2013). What this essentially means is that the focus of analysis is limited to the impact on the healthcare costs and patient health benefits, in terms of health related quality of life and quantity of life. Although health economists are increasing arguing for a broader "societal" perspective to be taken, whereby costs and benefits account for the wider impacts of health and care interventions (Neumann *et al.*, 2017; Walker *et al.*, 2019), the most common approach in practice continues to adopt a healthcare perspective (Kim *et al.*, 2020).

3.2 Generating QALYs

Moving from a CBA to a CEA economic evaluation framework requires a greater level of consideration as to how to measure and value benefits from health and care. Typically, it requires consideration of outcomes from interventions that account for the dual goal of capturing changes to quality and quantity of life. Otherwise, comparisons between interventions that only impact quality or quantity of life or both are not comparable for resource allocation purposes (Weinstein *et al.*, 2009).

The QALY has become the main outcome used to quantify the benefits of health and care interventions in economic evaluations. The idea of using QALYs was initially developed fifty years ago. The use of QALYs in healthcare decision-making has been driven by health economists, but also by a need in health and care to efficiently allocate scarce healthcare resources (MacKillop and Sheard, 2018).

QALYs represent patient benefits in a composite measure of health related quality of life, adjusted for the life years that health related quality of life was experienced. So if a person lives in a perfect health state with a quality of life score of 1 for a year, that person would have one QALY. Any gains in length of life are thus valued by the health related quality of life experienced during that period (Weinstein *et al.*, 2009).

Whilst the life years component of QALYs is relatively straightforward to calculate – from an analytical point of view, it is simply a case of whether or not someone is alive – the quality adjustment requires much more consideration. Here, the focus will be on the most commonly recommended approach for generating the quality adjustment in QALYs (Kennedy-Martin *et al.*, 2020).

Firstly, a health state measure/questionnaire is completed by patients. A common health state measure used in the generation of QALYs is the EQ-5D. EQ-5D measures health across five dimensions that looks to identify problems in mobility, self-care, usual activities, pain/discomfort and anxiety/depression (Devlin and Brooks, 2017). Patients complete the five EQ-5D questions before, during and after treatment to see how their health-related quality of life has changed as a result of treatment. Clinical trials, where patients receive different treatments for the same condition, is one way that allows for the cost-effectiveness between different interventions to be assessed.

The next step in generating QALYs is to assign *preferences* or *weights* or *values* to all possible health states. QALYs are anchored on a 0-1 *dead-perfect health* scale, whereby milder health states are likely to be closer to 1 and more severe health states closer to 0. Health states valued below zero are also technically possible on the QALY scale (Carr-Hill, 1989).

QALY weights tend to be assigned through general population surveys, where people are asked to give *stated preferences* for different health states over others (Weinstein *et al.*, 2009). There are a number of different options available for conducting such valuation exercises (Brazier *et al.*, 2017). The method used by NICE in England is the time trade-off method, whereby people are asked to choose between better health-related quality of life for a shorter quantity of life, compared to worse health-related quality of life for a longer time period (Dolan, 1995).

There are a number of reasons why health economists argue that general population surveys are conducted instead of specific patient valuations. General population valuation exercises allow for comparisons across a range of patient groups. It also allows members of the general population to have input into healthcare decisions for taxpayer funded healthcare, such as in England (Drummond *et al.*, 2015, p. 165). Another argument states that adopting a Rawlsian "veil of ignorance" approach allows for a more neutral stance across patient groups in the average estimate of generic health state values (Williams, 1996).

3.3 Using QALYs to aid decision-making

Once a value set for all possible health states is available for a health status measure (e.g. EQ-5D), this then acts as a new currency that allows for the assessment of the cost-effectiveness of new health interventions. A decision-maker can then assess if the cost of additional QALY gains in a patient group is *worth* it. Using QALYs in health and care decision-making raises many ethical and philosophical questions.[2]

Early applications of attempting to introduce the QALY into decision-making focused on producing league tables. Interventions that produced the lowest cost-per-QALY gained were placed at the top of the league table, with the idea that interventions would be funded as far down the league table as available funding and healthcare resources would allow. However, the ranking

---

[2]   See Nord (Nord, 1999) and Hausman (Hausman, 2015).

of some interventions over others highlighted some of the ethical challenges associated with using QALYs in decision-making. For example, the initial league table produced in the Oregon experiment in the United States led to higher priority for minor health conditions (e.g. tooth capping) over life-saving interventions (e.g. appendectomy) (Hadorn, 1991).

A more indirect approach is now more commonly seen in healthcare decision-making when using QALYs. This is where a cost-per-QALY gain threshold a decision-maker is willing to pay acts as the cut off for what is likely to be deemed a cost-effective use of healthcare resources. In England, a threshold of £20,000–30,000 per QALY gain is considered by NICE as a cost-effective use of healthcare resources (NICE, 2018). This means that if an intervention can produce additional QALYs for less than the cost-per-QALY threshold value (i.e. less than £20,000 per QALY gain), it is considered cost-effective. Extenuating circumstances are required for approval with a cost-effectiveness of between £20,000–30,000 per QALY gain. A health technology with a cost-per-QALY above £30,000 is less likely to be recommended for funding by NICE (Dakin et al., 2015).

The exact origin of this arbitrary £20,000–£30,000 NICE cost-effectiveness threshold in England is not precisely known. Early estimates for cost-effectiveness in the United States were benchmarked on the cost of renal dialysis in the 1970s, which were estimated to be around $50,000 per QALY gain (Neumann et al., 2014). This number roughly translates to the £20,000–£30,000 threshold used by NICE, when applying long-term currency conversion rates between the United States and the UK.

4   An alternative to QALYs based on the Capability Approach

From a public policy perspective, an outcome like QALYs, that are focused on health-related quality of life, makes it difficult to compare benefits across other sectors in society and so limits comparisons to a healthcare budget. This is increasingly problematic as health and care systems continue to expand the services they provide, such as the growing trend of *social prescribing*, including the "cycling on prescription" intervention to tackle obesity in England (DfT, 2020b).

QALYs represent a shift away from standard approaches to welfare assessment in economics. QALYs and the Disability Adjusted Life Years (DALYs) – a similar measure to QALYs that are typically used in CEA in low- and middle-income countries (Brazier et al., 2017, p. 303) – draw *post hoc* theoretical justification from Amartya Sen's critique of welfare economics assessment to support a shift away from the sole focus on utility (Culyer, 1989; Murray and Acharya, 1997).

Amartya Sen, a nobel prize winning economist and philosopher, dedicated much of his research to the role of standard welfare economics assessment in judging how "good" or "well" individuals are in society. His ideas have offered a compelling critique of economic analysis that limits such assessment to an individual's "utility", with the social welfare function of maximising utility likely to miss out important factors in the comparative assessment of wellbeing across society. He argued for a broadening of focus from individual's utility to also consider the person's capability to live a life they have reason to value (Sen, 1993).[3]

Sometimes referred to as extra-welfarism, proponents of QALYs and DALYs drew on Sen's work on functionings and capabilities to move away from a sole reliance on individual utility assessment. Yet, Sen's Capability Approach does not limit functionings assessment to health-related functionings. Sen also argued that focusing on functionings alone may be an insufficient assessment of a person's wellbeing without also assessing their capability to function across valuable different aspects of life (Sen, 1993). Therefore, extra-welfarism as currently applied in health economic evaluation is a limited interpretation of the Capability Approach in practice (Brouwer *et al.*, 2008).

4.1 Capability measures

An alternative application of extra-welfarism that more closely follows Sen's broader evaluative space has been developed. A number of capability measures have been developed over the past decade for different purposes across health and care settings (Helter *et al.*, 2020). Capability measures, such as the ICECAP capability measures (Al-Janabi *et al.*, 2012; Coast *et al.*, 2008a; Sutton and Coast, 2014), exhibit similar generic features to health state measures in that they allow for comparison across different patient groups to aid resource allocation decision-making across health and care. Capability measures have been recommended in economic evaluations for interventions in social care in England (NICE, 2016) and long-term care in the Netherlands (Zorginstituut Nederland, 2016), where QALYs have been recognised as being too narrowly focused on health to fully capture the benefits of interventions in these areas.

4.2 Measuring and valuing capabilities

Capability measures attempt to broaden the quality of life space captured in such tools by measuring capability directly. Attributes on the ICECAP

---

[3] See chapter by Ubels for further information on Sen's Capability Approach.

measures, for example, tend to be broad to allow respondents draw from a number of influences that might impact on their quality of life. For instance, the stability attribute on the ICECAP-A, worded as "feeling settled and secure", aims to cover not only health considerations, but also employment and finances, home and surroundings, friendships and family groups, and a strong belief system (Al-Janabi *et al.*, 2012). Indeed, for the ICECAP-A and ICECAP-O, the word *health* does not feature in the description of the attributes. Studies have shown associations between ICECAP attributes with physical and mental health measures (Afentou and Kinghorn, 2020; Proud *et al.*, 2019).

Measuring quality of life in terms of health or capability raises a similar challenge in that there is no gold standard measurement available for either concept (Streiner *et al.*, 2015). Therefore, different measurement tools place greater emphasis on certain areas over others depending on the population under consideration or the value judgements made by the respective measure developers (Pickles *et al.*, 2019; Richardson *et al.*, 2015). For instance, the attributes on the ICECAP measures were developed using qualitative research methods to identify the most important capabilities with members of the general public using semi-structured interviews. Other capability measures primarily rely on a pre-existing philosophical list of central human capabilities (Nussbaum, 2011, p. 33–34) to decide what items to capture on their measurement tool (Helter *et al.*, 2020).

A challenging aspect of implementing capability measures in economic evaluation is the role of valuing the relative importance of capabilities. Many of those who advocate a capabilities perspective reject any role of individuals preferences in deciding how to allocate resources, as Sen's critique of welfare economics emphasised the over-reliance of people's preferences in reaching decisions to pursue socially optimal policies (Robeyns, 2017). The default position in capabilities research is to treat all capabilities equally, with some arguing that capabilities cannot be traded off between one another (Simon *et al.*, 2013). Even though this argument provides an ideological departure from welfare economics, it does not necessarily provide helpful information to decision-makers where they have a choice of policies that prioritise some capabilities, and different people's capabilities, over others. However well-meaning attempts are to take a neutral stance where all capabilities are valued equally, such a position will still have implications if such measures are then used to aid decision-making concerning the allocation of scarce resources (Greco, 2018).

One valuation methodology that has been argued to link closely with Sen's critique of preferences, yet still allow for individual choices, is known as best-worst scaling. Best-worst scaling takes into account the extremes of people's preferences in terms of their most preferred and least preferred outcomes from a larger set of options. This valuation approach is based on random utility theory (Louviere *et al.*, 2015).

Best-worst scaling methodology therefore relaxes some of the strict preference assumptions made in stated preference studies that are used to generate QALYs; these instead rely on complete (or "transitive") preference ordering (Dagsvik, 2013). Another key advantage of best-worst scaling is that it is a relatively straightforward valuation task for people to complete. It allows people to participate who may be unable to otherwise (Bailey *et al.*, 2019).

4.3 Using capability measures to aid decision-making

A shift to valuing capabilities instead of health could also result in a change in how patient groups and condition severity are considered in economic evaluation. A multi-country study looking at the relative impacts of health and capability across seven different health conditions indicated that moving from a health to a capability focus would lead to priorities shifting towards mental health conditions, and interventions that improved severe and moderate health conditions compared to mild conditions (Mitchell *et al.*, 2015a).

One of Sen's seminal contributions was made when he posed and explored the following question – "the equality of what?" – meaning what areas in life are we trying to equalise across individuals to improve social welfare (Sen, 1992). Although Sen only mentioned it in a footnote in one of his contributions, he also stated that another important question to address is "the efficiency of what?" (Sen, 1993) – that is what are we trying to produce the most of at least cost to improve social welfare. This question has resulted in a relative shortage of research compared to important equality contributions that have been made in the Capability Approach (Robeyns, 2017). Nonetheless, one of the main contributions to this latter question has been made in health economic evaluations.

As with QALYs, decisions are required to be made about what the objective might be when measuring capabilities. Adopting the maximisation rule from welfare economics may not be an appropriate objective when trying to implement a broader application of the Capability Approach in economic evaluation (Coast, 2009). Indeed, there is growing recognition of the need for a sole focus on QALY maximisation to change in health economic evaluation, as it does not effectively deal with the dual public health policy goals of increasing population health and reducing health inequalities; these goals do not necessarily correlate with one another (Cookson *et al.*, 2017).

"Sufficient capability" is an attempt to focus on both societal wellbeing and inequalities of capabilities, by shifting the quality of life emphasis from health to capability, and the policy objective from maximisation to a decent or sufficient level of capability wellbeing (Mitchell *et al.*, 2015b). There are a number of different interpretations of what a sufficientarian objective actually entails (Fourie and Rid, 2017). For clarity, a shift to sufficient capability here prioritises the maximisation of capabilities only up to a level deemed sufficient and is consistent with other applications of the Capability Approach in practice (Mitchell *et al.*, 2017).

How to decide what a sufficient level of capability might be requires addressing when moving away from absolute maximisation. Deliberative research with the general public in England suggests that society would deem a sufficient level of capability on the ICECAP-A at the second highest level across all attributes for the purposes of public health and social care resource allocation decisions (Kinghorn, 2019). There are four levels on each of the five ICECAP-A attributes ranging from full capability, a lot of capability, a little capability and no capability (Al-Janabi *et al.*, 2012). Applying this sufficient capability threshold at "a lot" of capability means that any improvement in capability from "a lot" to "full" capability is not valued for public policy resource allocation purposes (Mitchell *et al.*, 2015b).

Using sufficient capability as the objective allows for the generation of Years of Sufficient Capability (YSC), whereby 1 YSC is equal to one year in a sufficient level of capability and 0 YSC is no capability across all capability states (Mitchell *et al.*, 2015b). To use YSC in decision-making, like QALYs, there is a requirement to establish how much a decision-maker or society is willing to pay for a YSC gain.[4] As well as shifting quality of life measurement from health to capability, a shift from maximisation to a sufficient capability objective could influence what interventions are considered a cost-effective use of health and care resources (Goranitis *et al.*, 2017).

Another consideration over the use of the current economic evaluation framework is that it treats what people value (e.g. generic health states) and how much they value it (using a single population valuation survey) the same irrespective of where individuals find themselves on the life-course. Ongoing research is looking to implement a new economic evaluation framework that allows for multiple capability measures to be used in aiding decision-making across the life-course (Coast, 2019). A life-course approach poses additional challenges when conducting economic evaluation, such as what measure or measures to use to fully capture the changes in quality of life at different stage of life (Mitchell *et al.*, 2020).

5 Summary

The discipline of economics is also known as the study of choice (Bishai and Rochaix, 2020).The choices that need to be made by policymakers in health and care can make economics, what some refer to as *the dismal science,* look even

---

[4]   See chapter by Himmler in this publication for ways this could be done.

more sombre. However, such decisions are required when healthcare resources are constrained, and choices need to be made over what treatments and patients to prioritise.

This chapter has highlighted the choices health economists have made to inform such decisions. An alternative way health economists can inform those decisions is proposed that (1) broadens the quality of life focus from health functionings to capabilities, and (2) moves from a health maximisation objective to one that prioritises getting individuals to a decent or sufficient level of capability (Mitchell *et al.*, 2015b). It is important for decision-makers to recognise that their choice of using QALYs or capability measures or any other measurement tool to aid resource allocation in health and care, will have an impact on what type of interventions and patient groups are prioritised under their remit (Mitchell *et al.*, 2015a).

Acknowledgements: I am grateful for the generous time countless numbers of people have given me over the years on topics covered in this chapter. In particular, conferences at the Human Development and Capability Association (HDCA), the International Health Economics Association (iHEA), the European Health Economics Association (EuHEA), and the UK Health Economists' Study Group (HESG); as well as journal clubs: Health Economics Unit (HEU) at the University of Birmingham, UK, King's Health Economics (KHE) at King's College London, and Health Economics Bristol (HEB) at the University of Bristol, UK; have all been very helpful. A previous version of this chapter was peer reviewed by Jordan Parsons, Jan Schildmann, and Jürgen Zerth. This chapter also benefitted from many fruitful discussions at the VALUEMED conference held in Fürth, Germany, in September 2019. Writing of this book chapter was supported by a Wellcome Investigator Award (PI: Joanna Coast): 205384/Z/16/Z.

References

Afentou, N. and Kinghorn, P. (2020), "A Systematic Review of the Feasibility and Psychometric Properties of the ICEpop CAPability Measure for Adults and Its Use So Far in Economic Evaluation", *Value in Health*, Vol. 23 No. 4, pp. 515–526.

Al-Janabi, H., Flynn T. N. and Coast, J. (2012), "Development of a self-report measure of capability wellbeing for adults: the ICECAP-A", *Quality of Life Research*, Vol. 21 No. 1, pp. 167–176.

Arrow, K. J. (1963), "Uncertainty and the Welfare Economics of Medical Care", *The American Economic Review*, Vol. 53 No. 5, pp. 941–973.

Bailey, C., Kinghorn, P., Hewison, A., Radcliffe, C., Flynn, T. N., Huynh, E. and Coast, J. (2019), "Hospice patients' participation in choice experiments to value supportive care outcomes", *BMJ Supportive & Palliative Care*, Vol. 9 No. 4, e37.

Bishai, D. and Rochaix, L. (2020), "The Meliorist Project in health economics", *Health Economics*, Vol. 29 No. 5, pp. 537–539.

Brazier, J. and Tsuchiya, A. (2015), "Improving cross-sector comparisons: going beyond the health-related QALY", *Applied Health Economics and Health Policy*, Vol. 13 No. 6, pp. 557–565.

Brazier, J., Ratcliffe, J., Salomon, J. A. and Tsuchiya, A. (2017), *Measuring and Valuing Health Benefits for Economic Evaluation*, 2nd ed., Oxford University Press, Oxford, UK.

Brouwer, W. B. F., Culyer, A. J., van Exel, N. J. A. and Rutten, F. F. H. (2008), "Welfarism vs. extra-welfarism", *Journal of Health Economics*, Vol. 27 No. 2, pp. 325–338.

Caro, J. J., Nord, E., Siebert, U., McGuire, A., McGregor, M., Henry, D., de Pouvourville, G., Atella, V. and Kolominsky-Rabas, P. (2010), "The efficiency frontier approach to economic evaluation of health-care interventions", *Health Economics*, Vol. 19 No. 10, pp. 1117–1127.

Carr-Hill, R. A. (1989), "Assumptions of the QALY procedure", *Social Science & Medicine*, Vol. 29 No. 3, pp. 469–477.

Coast, J. (2004), "Is economic evaluation in touch with society's health values?", *BMJ*, Vol. 329 No. 7476, pp. 1233–1236.

Coast, J. (2009), "Maximisation in extra-welfarism: A critique of the current position in health economics", *Social Science & Medicine*, Vol. 69 No. 5, pp. 786–792.

Coast, J. (2019), "Assessing capability in economic evaluation: a life course approach?", *The European Journal of Health Economics*, Vol. 20 No. 6, pp. 779–784.

Coast, J., Flynn, T. N., Natarajan, L., Sproston, K., Lewis, J., Louviere, J. J. and Peters, T. J. (2008a), "Valuing the ICECAP capability index for older people", *Social Science & Medicine*, Vol. 67 No. 5, pp. 874–882.

Coast, J., Smith R. and Lorgelly, P. (2008b), "Should the capability approach be applied in health economics?", *Health Economics*, Vol. 17 No. 6, pp. 667–670.

Coast, J., Smith, R. D. and Lorgelly, P. (2008c), "Welfarism, extra-welfarism and capability: the spread of ideas in health economics", *Social Science & Medicine*, Vol. 67 No. 7, pp. 1190–1198.

Cookson, R. (2005), "QALYs and the capability approach", *Health Economics*, Vol. 14 No. 8, pp. 817–829.

Cookson, R., Mirelman, A. J., Griffin, S., Asaria, M., Dawkins, B., Norheim, O. F., Verguet, S. and Culyer, A. J. (2017), "Using cost-effectiveness analysis to address health equity concerns", *Value in Health*, Vol. 20 No. 2, pp. 206–212.

Culyer, A. J. (1989), "The normative economics of health care finance and provision", *Oxford Review of Economic Policy*, Vol. 5 No. 1, pp. 34–58.

Dagsvik, J. K. (2013), "Making Sen's capability approach operational: a random scale framework", *Theory and Decision*, Vol. 74 No. 1, pp. 75–105.

Dakin, H., Devlin, N., Feng, Y., Rice, N., O'Neill, P. and Parkin, D. (2015), "The Influence of Cost-Effectiveness and Other Factors on NICE decisions", *Health Economics*, Vol. 24 No. 10, pp. 1256–1271.

Devlin, N. J. and Brooks, R. (2017), "EQ-5D and the EuroQol Group: Past, Present and Future", *Applied Health Economics and Health Policy*, Vol. 15 No. 2, pp. 127–137.

DfT (2017), *Airport Capacity in the South East: Moving Britain Ahead. Updated Appraisal Report*, Deparment for Transport (DfT), London.

DfT (2020a), *Full Business Case: High Speed 2 Phase One*, Department for Transport (DfT), London.

DfT (2020b), *Gear Change: A bold vision for cycling and walking*, Department for Transport (DfT), London.

Dolan, P. (1995), "Modeling Valuations for EuroQol Health States", *Medical Care*, Vol. 35 No. 11, pp. 1095–1108.

Drummond, M. F., Sculpher, M. J., Claxton, K., Stoddart, G. L. and Torrance, G. W. (2015), *Methods for the Economic Evaluation of Health Care Programmes*, 4th ed., Oxford University Press, Oxford, UK.

Ekelund, R. B. (1968), "Jules Dupuit and the Early Theory of Marginal Cost Pricing", *Journal of Political Economy*, Vol. 76 No. 3, pp. 462–471.

Fourie, C. and Rid, A. (2017), *What is enough? Sufficiency, justice and health*, Oxford University Press, New York.

Garrison, L. P., Neumann, P. J., Willke, R. J., Basu, A., Danzon, P. M., Doshi, J. A., Drummond, M. F., Lakdawalla, D. N., Pauly, M. K., Phelps, C. E., Ramsey, S. D., Towse, A. and Weinstein, M. C. (2018) "A Health Economics Approach to US Value Assessment Frameworks – Summary and Recommendations of the ISPOR Special Task Force Report [7]", *Value in Health*, Vol. 21 No. 2, pp. 161–165.

Goranitis, I., Coast, J., Day, E., Copello, A., Freemantle, N. and Frew, E. (2017), "Maximizing health or sufficient capability in economic evaluation? A methodological experiment of treatment for drug addiction", *Medical Decision Making*, Vol. 37 No. 5, pp. 498–511.

Greco, G. (2018), "Setting the Weights: The Women's Capabilities Index for Malawi", *Social Indicators Research*, Vol. 135, pp. 457–478.

Hadorn, D. C. (1991), "Setting Health Care Priorities in Oregon: Cost-effectiveness Meets the Rule of Rescue", *JAMA*, Vol. 265 No. 17, pp. 2218–2225.

Hauck, K., Morton, A., Chalkidou, K., Chi, Y., Culyer, A., Levin, C., Meacock, R., Over, M., Thomas, R., Vassall, A., Verguet, S. and Smith, P. C. (2019), "How can we evaluate the cost-effectiveness of health system strengthening? A typology and illustrations", *Social Science & Medicine*, Vol. 220, pp. 141–149.

Hausman, D. M. (2015), *Valuing health: well-being, freedom and suffering*, Oxford University Press, New York.

Helter, T. M., Coast, J., Łaszewska, A., Stamm, T. and Simon, J. (2020), "Capability instruments in economic evaluations of health-related interventions: a comparative review of the literature", *Quality of Life Research*, Vol. 29, pp. 1433–1464.

Jones, A. M. (2020), *The Oxford Encyclopedia of Health Economics*, Oxford University Press, Oxford, UK.

Karimi, M. and Brazier, J. (2016), "Health, health-related quality of life, and quality of life: what is the difference?", *Pharmacoeconomics*, Vol. 34, pp. 645–649.

Kennedy-Martin, M., Slaap, B., Herdman, M., van Reenen, M., Kennedy-Martin, T., Greiner, W., Busschbach, J. and Boye, K. S. (2020), "Which multi-attribute utility instruments are recommended for use in cost-utility analysis? A review of national health technology assessment (HTA) guidelines", *The European Journal of Health Economics*, doi: https://doi.org/10.1007/s10198-020-01195-8.

Kim, D. D., Silver, M. C., Kunst, N., Cohen, J. T., Ollendorf, D. A. and Neumann, P. J. (2020), "Perspective and Costing in Cost-Effectiveness Analysis, 1974–2018", *PharmacoEconomics*, doi: https://doi.org/10.1007/s40273-020-00942-2

Kinghorn, P. (2019), "Using deliberative methods to establish a sufficient state of capability well-being for use in decision-making in the contexts of public health and social care", *Social Science & Medicine*, Vol. 240, 112546.

KPMG (2018), *Temple Island Arena: Value for Money Assessment*, Bristol City Council, Bristol, UK.

Louviere, J. J., Flynn, T. N. and Marley, A. A. J. (2015), *Best-Worst Scaling: Theory, Methods and Applications*, Cambridge University Press, Cambridge, UK.

MacKillop, E. and Sheard, S. (2018), "Quantifying life: Understanding the history of Quality-Adjusted Life-Years (QALYs)", *Social Science & Medicine*, Vol. 211, pp. 359–366.

McIntosh, E., Clarke, P. M., Frew, E. J. and Louviere, J. J. (2010), *Applied Methods of Cost-Benefit Analysis in Health Care*, Oxford University Press, Oxford, UK.

Mitchell, P. M., Al-Janabi, H., Richardson, J., Iezzi, A. and Coast, J. (2015a), "The Relative Impacts of Disease on Health Status and Capability Wellbeing: A Multi-Country Study", *PloS ONE*, Vol. 10 No. 12, e0143590.

Mitchell, P. M., Roberts, T. E., Barton, P. M., and Coast, J. (2015b), "Assessing sufficient capability: a new approach to economic evaluation", *Social Science & Medicine*, Vol. 139, pp. 71–79.

Mitchell, P. M., Roberts, T. E., Barton, P. M. and Coast, J. (2017), "Applications of the Capability Approach in the Health Field: A Literature Review", *Social Indicators Research*, Vol. 133, pp. 345–371.

Mitchell, P. M., Caskey, F. J., Scott, J., Sanghera, S. and Coast, J. (2020), "Response process validity of three patient reported outcome measures for people requiring kidney care: a think-aloud study using the EQ-5D-5L, ICECAP-A and ICECAP-O", *BMJ Open*, Vol. 10 No. 5, e034569.

Morris, S., Devlin, N. and Parkin, D. (2007), *Economic Analysis in Health Care*, 1st ed., John Wiley & Sons Ltd., Chicester, England.

Murray, C. J. L. and Acharya, A. K. (1997), "Understanding DALYs", *Journal of Health Economics*, Vol. 16 No. 6, pp. 703–730.

Neumann, P. J., Cohen, J. T. and Weinstein, M. C. (2014), "Updating cost-effectiveness—the curious resilience of the \$50,000 per-QALY threshold", *New England Journal of Medicine*, Vol. 371 No. 9, pp. 796–797.

Neumann, P. J., Sanders, G. D., Russell, L. B., Siegel, J. E. and Ganiats, T. G. (2017), *Cost-Effectiveness in Health and Medicine*, 2nd ed., Oxford University Press, New York.

NICE (2013), *Guide to the methods of technology appraisal*, National Institute for Health and Care Excellence (NICE), London.

NICE (2016), *The social care guidance manual*, National Institute for Health and Care Excellence (NICE), London.

NICE (2018), *Developing NICE guidelines: the manual*, National Institute for Health and Care Excellence (NICE), London.

Nord, E. (1999), *Cost-Value Analysis in Health Care: Making Sense out of QALYs*, Cambridge University Press, Cambridge, UK.

Nussbaum, M. C. (2011), "Creating capabilities: the human development approach", Belknap Harvard, Cambridge, Massachusetts.

Pickles, K., Lancsar, E., Seymour, J., Parkin, D., Donaldson, C. and Carter, S. M. (2019), "Accounts from developers of generic health state utility instruments explain why they produce different QALYs: A qualitative study", *Social Science & Medicine*, Vol. 240, 112560.

Proud, L., McLoughlin, C. and Kinghorn, P. (2019), "ICECAP-O, the current state of play: a systematic review of studies reporting the psychometric properties and use of the instrument over the decade since its publication", *Quality of Life Research*, Vol. 28 No. 6, pp. 1429–1439.

Richardson, J., Iezzi, A. and Khan, M. A. (2015), "Why do multi-attribute utility instruments produce different utilities: the relative importance of the descriptive systems, scale and 'micro-utility' effects", *Quality of Life Research*, Vol. 24, pp. 2045–2053.

Robeyns, I. (2017), *Wellbeing, Freedom and Social Justice: The Capability Approach Re-Examined*, Open Book Publishers, Cambridge, UK.

Rowen, D., Zouraq, I. A., Chevrou-Severac, H. and van Hout, B. (2017), "International regulations and recommendations for utility data for health technology assessment." *Pharmacoeconomics* 35 (1):11–19.

Sen, A. (1992), *Inequality Reexamined*, Oxford University Press, Oxford, UK.

Sen, A. (1993), "Capability and Well-Being", in Nussbaum, M. C. and Sen, A. (Ed.), *The Quality of Life*, Oxford University Press, Oxford, UK, pp. 30–53.

Sen, A. (2002), "Health: perception versus observation", *BMJ*, Vol. 324 No. 7342, pp. 860–861.

Simon, J., Anand, P., Gray, A., Rugkåsa, J., Yeeles, K. and Burns, T. (2013), "Operationalising the capability approach for outcome measurement in mental health research", *Social Science & Medicine*, Vol. 98, pp. 187–196.

Streiner, D. L., Norman, G. R. and Cairney, J. (2015), *Health Measurement Scales: a practical guide to their development and use*, 5th ed., Oxford University Press, Oxford, UK.

Sutton, E. J. and Coast, J. (2014), "Development of a supportive care measure for economic evaluation of end-of-life care using qualitative methods", *Palliative Medicine*, Vol. 28 No. 2, pp. 151–157.

Taylor, R. S., Drummond, M. F., Salkeld, G. and Sullivan, S. D. (2004), "Inclusion of cost effectiveness in licensing requirements of new drugs: the fourth hurdle", *BMJ*, Vol. 329 No. 7472, pp. 972–975.

Walker, S., Griffin, S., Asaria, M., Tsuchiya, A. and Sculpher, M. (2019), "Striving for a societal perspective: a framework for economic evaluations when costs and effects fall on multiple sectors and decision makers." *Applied Health Economics and Health Policy*, Vol. 17 No. 5, pp. 577–590.

Weinstein, M. C., Torrance, G. and McGuire, A. (2009), "QALYs: The Basics", *Value in Health*, Vol. 12 S. 1, pp. S5–S9.

Williams, A. (1996), "QALYs and ethics: a health economist's perspective", *Social Science & Medicine*, Vol. 43 No. 12, pp. 1795–1804.

Wisløff, T., Hagen, G., Hamidi, V., Movik, E., Klemp, M. and Olsen, J. A. (2014), "Estimating QALY gains in applied studies: a review of cost-utility analyses published in 2010", *Pharmacoeconomics*, Vol. 32, pp. 367–375.

Zorginstituut Nederland (2016), *Guidelines for economic evaluations in healthcare*, Zorginstituut Nederland

The assessment of value in health economics: utility and capability

Jasper Ubels

Abstract

There is a discussion within the field of health economics about the appropriate informational base on which to assess value. One method to assess value in medical interventions is with the quality-adjusted life year (QALY). In the calculation of QALYs, the value of a life year is adjusted with a utility value. Multiple conceptualizations of utility exist. In one of these conceptualizations, utility represents a positive mental state; in another, utility reflects the preferences of individuals for certain things.

However, according to Nobel Laureate Amartya Sen, these conceptualizations of utility have limitations. Essentially, he argues that things might have an economic value beyond utility for a multitude of reasons. The first reason being that people might place value on their ability to choose between different alternatives beyond the availability of an alternative that maximizes an individual's utility, for the sake of choice itself. Second, individuals might choose things that go against their personal preferences for a variety of different motivations. The third reason is related to the positive mental health state conceptualization of utility. One particular problem with this conceptualization is that people adapt to limitations. This leads to individuals with severe disabilities reporting higher levels of subjective wellbeing than expected. In short, utility itself is too limited of a concept to use as the informational base for the assessment of value.

Instead, Sen argues that the value assessment should be based on the capabilities of individuals. Capabilities are understood as the freedom of individuals to do or to be. That what people are or are doing with their freedom, is called functionings. Sen argues that the use of capabilities as an informational base is preferred over utility and functioning. Namely, through measurement of capability, it is possible to measure all the alternative options available to an individual. This includes the utility derived from those options as well as the value of being able to choose between options. Furthermore, adaptation by individuals to limitations does not influence the assessment of value, since the informational base of capability is concerned with the freedom of individuals to do or be. Thus, by using capabilities as the informational base, it is possible to assess the value of medical interventions without the problems posed by using utility.

However, is the measurement of capabilities alone sufficient to assess value? Based on theoretical considerations by Fleurbay and Clark, as well as observational studies in patients affected by the locked-in syndrome, a medical condition in which a patient is aware but cannot communicate due to muscle paralysis, this chapter concludes that this is not the case. Capability, functioning and utility are all, when used individually, insufficient to estimate the value of a medical intervention. Instead, information about capability, functioning and utility needs to be combined for an appropriate assessment of the value of medical interventions.

Keywords: Capability approach, utility, outcome measurement, health technology assessment, value assessment, patient-reported outcomes

1 Introduction

This chapter will dive deeper into the theory underlying the assessment of value in the context of evaluating medical interventions.[1] Section one presents the informational base that is used to assess value in conventional health economics. *Informational base* refers to the kind of information used to assess value. In section two, the fundamental critique of conventional economics by Amartya Sen and his theory about the appropriate informational base on which to assess value are introduced. In section three, Sen's theory is scrutinized. The chapter concludes with the assertion that Sen's theory of the appropriate informational base of value and certain understandings of utility need to be combined to have a complete informational base on which assess value.

2 The informational base in conventional health economics

The QALY is a measure that combines information about both the length and the quality of life. QALYs are applied in the valuation of medical interventions by assessing the increase in life years as a result of a medical interventions along with the utility adjusted quality of each of those life years (Torrance, 1986).[2]

---

[1]   In the chapter by Mitchell in this publication, a general overview was provided how health economists conduct economic evaluations. Furthermore, it contained a general introduction in the theory and applications of the capability approach.

[2]   In the previous chapter by Mitchell, the use of questionnaires to estimate Quality Adjusted Life Years (QALYs) was explained.

The concept utility itself can be understood in a variety of different ways – for a discussion, see Sen (1985b) and Richardson (1994). In one conceptualization, utility is viewed as the happiness of an individual (Sen, 1985b). In this understanding, utility is a representation of a person's positive mental health state. The value of a medical intervention would be expressed by its effect on the happiness of an individual. Medical interventions that, for example, increase the happiness of an individual create utility, thus providing value.

An alternative way of looking at the utility value of something is by expressing utility in terms of the preferences of individuals. These preferences can be observed by the individuals' choice behaviour (Luce and Raiffa, 1958)[3]. From such observations, an *ordinal scale* can be generated. The following example illustrates how this works in practice. Take a set of snacks consisting of chocolate bars, lollipops, chewing gum and broccoli. From this set, you can observe an individual choosing a bar of cholate. In this case, it is possible to say that a chocolate bar has a higher utility compared to the lollipops, chewing gum, and broccoli.

However, based on this observation, it is not possible to attribute numerical values to this utility. By observing the choice of an individual, we can only know which snack is preferred over the other by that individual. We can thus create a ranking of the snacks in terms of utility. However, by doing so we only know the order of preferences for the snacks. We have no information about how much stronger the preference for one snack is over another.

In order to attribute numerical values to utility that represent the strength of a preference, a more sophisticated framework with further assumptions is necessary. In the context of the example presented above, it is possible to translate the preference of an individual for a certain type of snack into a numerical utility value assigned to that snack. By doing so, a *cardinal scale* is created. One way of eliciting these numerical values is by introducing a gamble, which might consists of two choices (Drummond *et al.*, 2015; Gafni, 1994): choice one is a certain probability of the individual eating a chocolate bar, let's say probability p is $p = 0.4$. This probability is coupled with the probability of not eating anything, which is $p = 0.6$. Choice two is eating broccoli. Then through an iterative process, it is possible to find that probability of eating chocolate compared to not eating something at all where someone is indifferent between choice one and choice two. This point could be at $p = 0.2$ of eating a chocolate bar (with an associated probability $p = 0.8$ of not eating anything). Then, it is possible to say that from a scale from 0, which means not eating anything at all, to 1, which is eating chocolate, broccoli has a utility value of 0.2. A similar exercise can be repeated separately for lollipops and

---

[3]   Known as the "expected utility hypothesis". For an excellent explanation of the axioms and assumptions underpinning this theory, see chapter two in the book Games and Decisions by Luce and Raiffa (1958, pp. 12–37).

chewing gum. This way, by using eating a chocolate bar and not eating anything as anchor points for a scale, it is possible to create a numerical scale for
the utility of eating broccoli, lollipops and chewing gum. This numerical scale
gives the numerical value of eating broccoli, lollipops and chewing gum on a
scale from eating nothing to eating chocolate. The above presented exercise is
called the "standard gamble".

An example of how the standard gamble is used in health economics is
illustrated by how utility values are generated for the EQ-5D (Rabin and Charro,
2001). The EQ-5D is a standardized instrument to assess the value of a medical
intervention. It measures health related quality of life and consists of five different health related domains: mobility, self-care, usual activities,
pain/discomfort and anxiety/depression. Per domain there are response categories representing different levels of health. For example, the domain
pain/discomfort contains response categories ranging from "I have extreme
pain or discomfort" to "I have no pain or discomfort". One standard approach
of using the EQ-5D is by measuring the change in the score of the different
domains of questionnaire in a group of people before and after a new medical
intervention is applied. This change is compared to the change in a control
group where a standard treatment is administered. These domain scores can be
translated into so-called utility values. The difference in the magnitude of
change of the domain scores between the group where the medical intervention is applied and the control group with a standard treatment is the utility
value of that medical intervention. This utility value is usually associated with
a timeframe, which is typically a year. In this way, the effect of a medical intervention on the quality of a life year is assessed and QALYs can be calculated.
But how are these utility values for domain scores generated? One method for
doing so is by applying the standard gamble exercise to translate domain
scores of the EQ-5D into utility values.

Domain of EQ5D	Level in domain
Mobility	I have some problems walking about
Self-Care	I am unable to wash or dress myself
Usual Activities	I have some problems with performing my usual activities
Pain / Discomfort	I have no pain or discomfort
Anxiety / Depression	I am not anxious or depressed

Table 1. Example of a health state based on the EQ5D.

A standard gamble exercise for the elicitation of utility values for the different
combinations of domain scores consists of presenting a sample of the population with a health state that is a combination of answer categories of these
domains. An exemplary health state can be found in table 1.

Then, participants are asked to either live in that health state for the rest of their lives, or choose the alternative option. This alternative option is to be immediately healthy for the rest of their lives, with a probability of dying. That point where the probability of becoming healthy immediately or die is equal to living in a certain health state for a number of years represents the utility value for that health state[4].

The theoretical framework on which the standard gamble is based is the von Neumann-Morgenstern theory of utility, otherwise known as expected utility theory (Gafni, 1994; Torrance, 1986). This theory is developed to explain how people should make rational decisions under uncertainty, while taking into account the strength of the preferences of individuals. It is important to be aware of the theoretical assumptions underlying the elicitation of preferences, because failure to meet one of the assumptions might result in the elicited preferences being invalid. One important assumption in the context of preference measurement is that the preferences themselves are assumed to be "complete" (Warren *et al.*, 2011). This means, that an individual knows what kind of options are available, and is able to provide a subjective value to those options, which are expressed when an individual makes a choice.

As with any framework, there are proponents and opponents discussing the merits and flaws of the use of expected utility theory to assess the value of things[5]. However, in the conventional health economic practice, utility plays an important role as the informational base for the assessment of value.

3 Broadening the informational base with the capability approach

3.1 *Amartya Sen and the capability approach*

In the previous section an introduction was given about the use of utility as the informational base on which value is assessed in the field of health economics. We also mentioned that there are critics of the use of utility. One of the most prominent criticists is Amartya Sen. Sen criticizes the methods used to elicit utility, but also argues that utility as an informational base to assess value is limited in the first place (Sen, 1985a).

---

[4]   Of course, other frames and methods can and are being used to elicit utility values in different contexts. See for an overview of the methods used in conventional health economics the book "Methods for the economic evaluation of health care programmes" by Drummond (2015).

[5]   See Richardson (1994) for a discussion of various utility elicitation methods. Furthermore, see Richardson (1994) and Luce and Raiffa (1958, pp. 12–37) for discussions about the tautological nature of utility in expected utility theory.

To best appreciate Sen's critique, it is necessary to understand his alternative theory that, amongst other things, justifies a broader informational base for the assessment of value. Sen calls this theory the capability approach. In this approach, Sen argues that the informational base that is used to evaluate the life of an individual should not be limited to what an individual is or does. Instead, the assessment of wellbeing should focus on *the freedom* of what an individual can be or can do (Sen, 1985a). The value of medical intervention can then, amongst other things, be based on its effects on the freedom of an individual. The benefits of extending the informational base for the assessment of value to the freedom of individuals is illustrated in the following example:

Imagine two individuals: Karla and Pierre. Both Karla and Pierre are losing weight. However, there is a difference between Karla and Pierre. Karla lives in an affluent area with enough possibilities to eat, but chooses to fast. Pierre lives in an impoverished area that is affected by famine and is starving. As a consequence, both Karla and Pierre are equally hungry because of their food intake. By only considering what Karla and Pierre are actually eating, it is impossible to say who is better off. However, when taking into account what Karla and Pierre *can* eat, it is clear that Karla is better off than Pierre.

In the context of the capability approach, the actual level of food intake by Karla and Pierre would be their functioning; the freedom to eat, a capability. By extending the informational base for the assessment of value to the capabilities of individuals, proponents of the capability approach argue that a more complete picture of the wellbeing of an individual can be assessed, which also results in an improved assessment of value of interventions aimed at increasing how well-off individuals are.

3.2 The advantages of using capability over utility

But what are the advantages of using capability as an informational base for the assessment of value over utility? One of the critiques of Sen on the use of expected utility is that things might have value beyond the preferences of individuals (Sen, 1985b). Take for example again, the scenario with the chocolate, the lollipop, chewing gum, and broccoli. Even if a person is only interested in eating chocolate, it is still possible that the mere ability to choose from the different snacks (or not eat anything at all) may lead to higher levels of wellbeing. In other words, if all the other snack options are taken away except for chocolate (which is possibly the preferred choice over the other snacks), one might still experience being worse off, since choice itself can be seen as part of life (Sen, 1993).

Additionally, by extending the evaluative space to capability, one takes into account the fact that people might choose things that might not be their immediate preference or create happiness (Sen, 1985b). For example, a father may choose to eat broccoli instead of chocolate, all the while preferring chocolate, in order to set a good example for his child. In this case, the choice is not only limited to the father's own interests, but also takes the interest of another into account. This contradicts the conclusions that are drawn from the utility elicitation methods presented in section one, since people value (and have reason to value) things beyond their own preferences and their personal happiness.

Furthermore, can we trust that people have complete preferences? It is very much possible that people are not aware of all the choice options available to them, and they might also be unable to have a value for each of these options. To illustrate these points in the context of the assessment of an individual's health, Sen (2002) compared the life expectancy of the United States and various states of India with the incidence of self-reported morbidity of the United States and those respective states of India. Self-reported morbidity is a way of assessing disease in a population, where you ask people what kind of diseases or symptoms of diseases they have. Sen observed that people who live in regions with *higher* levels of education, *better* medical care and *higher* life expectancy report *more* comorbidities. Vice versa, the inhabitants of regions with *lower* levels of education, *worse* medical care might and *lower* life expectancy report *less* comorbidities. Sen concluded, that relying on the self-reported information of people often results in misleading evaluations of the health of those people. Furthermore, it is also questionable if the self-reported preferences of individuals are a trustworthy source of information – see (Warren *et al.*, 2011) for a discussion regarding preference construction.

Moreover, when utility is understood as reflecting a positive mental health state, another problem appears: that of adaptation. According to Sen, people can be happy and consider themselves to be well off even under dire circumstances (Sen, 1985b). This adaptation phenomenon occurs because people can adapt to limitations in their capabilities. A practical example of this can be found in patients affected by the so called "locked-in syndrome" (LIS). Patients affected by LIS are severely impaired in their movement abilities, but are otherwise not severely cognitively impaired (Smith and Delargy, 2005). Patients affected by LIS can have a life expectancy of up to several decades (Laureys *et al.*, 2005). Patients can typically be divided in certain subgroups. These subgroups range from "incomplete" LIS, where patients have some rudimentary movement ability left, such as the movement of a foot or a finger, to complete LIS, where patients are completely unable to move, including movement of their eyes (Smith and Delargy, 2005).

Surprisingly, patients affected by LIS report reasonably high levels of subjective wellbeing (Bruno *et al.*, 2011; Rousseau *et al.*, 2015). Bruno *et al.* (2011) measured subjective wellbeing on an 11-point scale, with answers ranging from "as bad as in the worst period in my life" to "as well as in the best period in my life[6]". Despite their physical limitations, patients considered themselves to be well off. Furthermore, the patients' reported wellbeing remained stable over a longer period of time (Rousseau *et al.*, 2015). This observation is a defence for the assessment of the wellbeing of individuals in terms of their capabilities, as one could argue that even though the subjective wellbeing of patients affected by LIS is high, people without LIS are, nevertheless, better off. Thus, by looking at the disadvantages of using utility as the informational base on which to assess value and the advantages of focusing on capability, it seems that capabilities are a more appropriate informational base on which to assess value.

Finally, according to Sen, by assessing value in terms of capability, it is also possible to capture the utility that people derive from having that capability. For example, by evaluating the capability to eat certain snacks, one also includes the evaluation of the utility, since the evaluative space covers all the possible preferences of the individual, as well as the happiness derived from eating certain snacks (Sen, 1985a). Thus, capabilities are argued to be a sufficient informational base to assess value. Unfortunately, Sen does not provide an in depth explanation of how capability is related to utility, particularly in the context of utility conceptualized as a positive mental state. This lack of explanation has been considered a limitation of the capability approach (Clark, 2005).

4   The need to integrate utility and the capability approach

In the last section we discussed the limitations of this use of utility as an informational base for the assessment of value based on the work of Sen. Furthermore, we introduced the capability approach as an alternative theory which argues for the extending the informational base of the evaluation of value to the capabilities of individuals. This was followed up with a discussion of the advantages of extending the informational base of value to capability.

However, should it be concluded that capabilities are a sufficient informational base to assess value? The example of Karla and Pierre illustrates, of course, that the use of capability adds additional information beyond utility that we have reason to value. However, authors have pointed out the limitations of solely using capability as the informational base on which to assess value (Clark, 2005; Fleurbaey, 2006). According to Fleurbaey (2006), the hunger and fasting example does not show that capabilities themselves are a sufficient

---

[6]   Bruno *et al.* (2011) slightly adapted the so called Anamnestic Comparative Self-Assessment Scale, by changing the two optimal answer categories" from "the best period in my life" to "the best period prior to LIS".

base of information, but merely show the added benefit of extending the informational base to capability in the assessment of wellbeing. Fleurbaey (2006) argues that in order to show that the use of capabilities is sufficient, an alternative thought experiment is necessary. In this thought experiment, the capabilities of two individuals are the same, but due to the choices made by the individuals, the resulting functionings are different. If the result of this thought experiment shows that there is no difference in the level of wellbeing between these individuals, then we can conclude that capability is indeed a sufficient informational base.

For this thought experiment[7], we take two hypothetical individuals: Ronald and Norris. Ronald and Norris have very similar backgrounds. Both are college educated, middle-class men living with a small family in the same suburb. Also in terms of their capabilities, Ronald and Norris are similar. Near the houses of Norris and Ronald you can find a fast-food outlet. Here, there is a difference between Norris and Ronald. Norris decides to eat every day in this fast-food outlet, where Ronald only visits the outlet infrequently. Over the years, Norris' unhealthy choices have resulted in his having health issues, while Ronald remains fit, in part due to his choice to eat healthy food. In this case, Ronald and Norris achieve certain functionings, given the capabilities which they have and the choices they make within those capabilities. However, the functionings achieved are very different for Ronald and Norris. Given this, are Ronald and Norris equally well off? Fleurbaey (2006) argues that capabilities themselves are an insufficient informational base to answer this question. Instead, he proposes that the assessment of wellbeing should combine information about an individual's capabilities with information about the individual's achieved functionings, to get a full picture of the wellbeing of an individual. In the case of Ronald and Norris, you could then argue that in the end, Ronald is indeed better off, given that he does not have any health problems.

Is an informational base of value based on functioning and capability than sufficient? No, according to Clark (2005). Clark argues that the capability approach, as conceptualized by Sen, leaves too little space for one understanding of utility to be assessed: that of mental states that people have reason to value (such as happiness or life satisfaction). By limiting the capability approach to the measurement of capability and functioning, as argued by Fleurbaey (2006), it is possible that valuable aspects of utility are not measured.

To illustrate this, we can revisit the snack example. Recall earlier in this chapter the example of the capability of eating a snack as the informational base to assess the value of that snack. Based on this example it was argued, that by evaluating the capability of eating a snack, it is also possible to capture the utility derived from the functioning of eating a snack. Now imagine that due to

---

[7]   Example is based on example introduced by Fleurbay (2006).

a pandemic, Karla and Pierre are required to stay quarantined at home for two months and are to refrain from any kind of human contact. Now imagine that the only food is available in Karla's and Pierre's homes are the snacks presented earlier in the chapter: chocolate, a lollipop, chewing gum and broccoli. Depending on the preferences of Karla and Pierre, the first couple of hours in quarantine be problematic with these types of food. In fact, they might enjoy the excuse to eat one of the snacks presented above, given that they are not able to access other types of food. However, after a while, Karla feels frustrated about eating the same snacks repeatedly. This is problematic for Karla, since due to the pandemic people are required to stay at home for two months and are not allowed to go out or meet with anyone. Thus, Karla and Pierre must keep eating these snacks to stay alive. Pierre, on the other hand, is happy to continue eating such snacks, especially due to his passion for chocolate.

How is the value of the snacks assessed in terms of capability, functioning and utility? In terms of capabilities, Karla's and Pierre's situation has not changed from the first day of quarantine to the last, since they still have a variety of snacks to choose from. Furthermore, their capabilities are comparable, since they are both forced to stay at home. Also in terms of their functionings, there has not been a change because by eating the snacks, Karla and Pierre always achieve a similar level of functioning. However, one difference can be identified. The difference between Karla and Pierre is their utility, understood as a positive mental health state or the fulfilment of desire. Karla feels significantly worse than Pierre, which is not captured by assessing their capabilities or their functionings. Thus, only the informational base of utility manages to capture the difference in wellbeing between Karla and Pierre in their two months of quarantine.

For a real-world example, consider again patients affected by LIS. As was noted before, patients affected by LIS generally experience good levels of wellbeing, especially considering their limitations in capability (and as a consequence their functioning) (Bruno *et al.*, 2011; Rousseau *et al.*, 2015). Still, it is interesting to note that within the patient group affected by LIS, there is a large variation in the levels of subjective wellbeing. Recall that in these studies, the subjective wellbeing of the patients was assessed by letting people assess their own lives on a scale ranging from the worst period in their lives to the best period in their lives (Bruno *et al.*, 2011). Even under similar circumstances, in terms of capability and given the limitations due to LIS, two subgroups can be identified. One of these groups report "good" levels of subjective wellbeing, while the other groups reports "bad" levels of subjective wellbeing. Bruno *et al.* (2011) reported a significant difference between the two groups in terms of time spent in LIS (with shorter time relating to lower levels of subjective wellbeing), lack of recovery in speech, depression, anxiety, perceived ability to participate in recreational activities, the perceived adequate level of mobility in the patients community, perceived ability to cope with live events, attitude towards resuscitation in case of cardiac arrest, suicidal thoughts and intended euthanasia by patients.

Particularly a lack of recovery in speech, an inability to participate in recreational activities, and the perception of having an inadequate level of mobility in their community can be seen as factors that limit the capability of patients affected by LIS. These factors severely limit the capability of patients to participate in a variety of capabilities that they have reason to value. Still, the authors noted that the explanatory power of the total combination of variables included in their analysis (including ones that showed no significant difference between the group with good levels of subjective wellbeing and bad levels of subjective wellbeing[8]) only explain a limited amount of the variance in the subjective wellbeing of the patients (38%)[9]. This practical example shows that the subjective wellbeing of an individual is not assessed if you focus on evaluating only the capability and functioning of individuals.

5   Conclusion

In summary, capability, functioning, and utility, in terms of mental state, taken separately, may be insufficient informational bases for the assessment of value. Instead, each bring their own kind of information to the table, which combined creates a complete picture of an individual's wellbeing. This has the consequence that in order to get a complete picture of the value of a medical intervention, information is needed about: 1) how the medical intervention influences the capability of an individual; 2) the influence of the medical intervention on what an individual does with that capability; and 3) how the individual experiences his or her capability. How can an informational base which is a combination of constructs be measured in the context of assessing the value of medical interventions? One way of measuring this is through the use of questionnaires with broad domains that reflect what people value. These question-

---

[8]   These are variables related to perceived adequacy of mobility in a variety of different contexts, comfortability of fulfilling self-care needs, ability to participate in work and social activities, ability to fulfil role in family needs, conformability with personal relationships, conformability with being in company of others and pain.

[9]   The dependent variable in this regression is the self-assessment of good life, with the independent variables: lack of recovery in speech, depression, anxiety, perceived ability to participate in recreational activities, the perceived adequate level of mobility in the patients community, perceived ability to cope with live events, attitude towards resuscitation in case of cardiac arrest, suicidal thoughts, intended euthanasia by patients, variables related to perceived adequacy of mobility in a variety of different contexts, comfortability of fulfilling self-care needs, ability to participate in work and social activities, ability to fulfil role in family needs, conformability with personal relationships, conformability with being in company of others and pain.

naires should be developed together with the people for which medical interventions are developed to improve their wellbeing.[10]

How then, can we know how much a combination of capabilities, functioning and utility is worth? Or should monetary values even be assigned? These remain open questions.[11]

References

Bruno, M.-A., Bernheim, J. L., Ledoux, D., Pellas, F., Demertzi, A. and Laureys, S. (2011), "A survey on self-assessed well-being in a cohort of chronic locked-in syndrome patients: happy majority, miserable minority", *BMJ open*, Vol. 1 No. 1, p. e000039.

Clark, D. A. (2005), "Sen's capability approach and the many spaces of human well-being", *The Journal of Development Studies*, Vol. 41 No. 8, pp. 1339–1368.

Drummond, M. F., Sculpher, M. J., Claxton, K., Stoddart, G. L. and Torrance, G. W. (2015), *Methods for the economic evaluation of health care programmes*. Oxford University Press.

Fleurbaey, M. (2006), "Capabilities, functionings and refined functionings", *Journal of Human Development*, Vol. 7 No. 3, pp. 299–310.

Gafni, A. (1994), "The standard gamble method: what is being measured and how it is interpreted", *Health Services Research*, Vol. 29 No. 2, p. 207.

Laureys, S., Pellas, F., Van Eeckhout, P., Ghorbel, S., Schnakers, C., Perrin, F., Berre, J., Faymonville, M.-E., Pantke, K.-H. and Damas, F. (2005), "The locked-in syndrome: what is it like to be conscious but paralyzed and voiceless?", *Progress in Brain Research*, Vol. 150, pp. 495–611.

Luce, R. D. and Raiffa, H. (1958), "Games and decisions: Introduction and critical survey", Wiley New York, pp. 12–37.

Rabin, R. and Charro, F. d. (2001), "EQ-SD: a measure of health status from the EuroQol Group", *Annals of Medicine*, Vol. 33 No. 5, pp. 337–343.

Richardson, J. (1994), "Cost utility analysis: what should be measured?", *Social Science & Medicine*, Vol. 39 No.1, pp. 7–21.

Rousseau, M.-C., Baumstarck, K., Alessandrini, M., Blandin, V., De Villemeur, T. B. and Auquier, P. (2015), "Quality of life in patients with locked-in syndrome: Evolution over a 6-year period", *Orphanet Journal of Rare Diseases*, Vol. 10 No.1, p. 88.

Sen, A. (1985a), *Commodities and Capabilities*. Amsterdam: North Holland.

Sen, A. (1985b), "Well-being, agency and freedom: The Dewey lectures 1984", *The Journal of Philosophy*, Vol. 82 No.4, pp. 187–190.

Sen, A. (1993), "Capability and Well-Being", in Nussbaum, M. and Sen, A. (Ed.) *The Quality of Life*, ed., Oxford University Press, New York.

Sen, A. (2002), "Health: perception versus observation: self reported morbidity has severe limitations and can be extremely misleading". *British Medical Journal Publishing Group*, Vol. 324, pp. 860–861.

---

[10] Examples of such questionnaires were introduced and discussed in the chapter by Mitchell in this publication.

[11] Possible answers to these questions are explored in the next chapter of this publication by Himmler, which focuses on methods for eliciting monetary values for capabilities.

Smith, E. and Delargy, M. (2005), "Locked-in syndrome", *British Medical Journal Publishing Group*, Vol. 330 No. 7488, pp. 406–409.

Torrance, G. W. (1986), 'Measurement of health state utilities for economic appraisal: a review', *Journal of Health Economics*, Vol. 5 No. 1, pp. 1–30.

Warren, C., McGraw, A. P. and Van Boven, L. (2011), "Values and preferences: defining preference construction", *Wiley Interdisciplinary Reviews: Cognitive Science*, Vol. 2 No. 2, pp. 193–205.

Estimating the monetary value of health: why and how[1]

Sebastian Himmler

Abstract

The efficient allocation of scarce health care resources is an important but difficult task. Health economic evaluation, and more specifically, cost-effectiveness analysis, can be a helpful tool for informing these allocation decisions. While some consider comparing costs to health outcomes as an impossible trade-off, it is defensible if made on a collective level, and considering that in a resource constraint setting, costs just quantify what care/benefits need to be sacrificed by others. If one accepts the cost-effectiveness framework, one also accepts its decision rule, which states that a treatment is considered cost-effective if the ratio of cost per QALY is lower than a certain threshold, which is oriented either on what society is willing to pay for a QALY or on the opportunity costs of displaced care. This decision rule implies the necessity for obtaining monetary estimates of the value of a QALY. In previous research, this was mainly attempted by using two conceptually different approaches. First, and more recently, estimates of an opportunity cost based threshold were calculated based on the marginal returns to health care spending, with applications in the UK, Spain, the Netherlands and Sweden. A much larger branch of literature obtained estimates of the societal monetary valuation of a QALY. This was either based on the value of a statistical life (or prevented fatality), obtained through revealed or stated preferences, or on the societal willingness to pay for certain health gains using stated preferences techniques such as contingent valuation willingness to pay experiments or discrete choice experiments. The estimates of the monetary value of a QALY that were obtained are context and approach depended, and also can differ considerably if a similar approach is used in the same context. This chapter will outline an additional

---

[1] Parts of this chapter contain results from two articles by the author:
1. Himmler, S., van Exel, J., Brouwer, W. (2020), "Estimating the monetary value of health and capability well-being applying the well-being valuation approach.", *European Journal of Health Economics* https://doi.org/10.1007/s10198-020-01231-7.
2. Himmler S., Stöckel J., van Exel, J., Brouwer, W. (2020), "The Value of Health – Empirical Issues when Estimating the Monetary Value of a QALY Based on Well-Being Data.", *SOEPpapers on Multidisciplinary Panel Data Research,* 1101. https://www.econstor.eu/handle/10419/224090

alternative approach for estimating the monetary societal valuation of a QALY: the well-being valuation approach. This approach is not strictly based on either stated nor revealed preferences, and entails using regression analysis and observational data. Using life satisfaction (or SWB) as proxy for overall utility, the marginal rate of substitution of the well-being impact of income and health is calculated to obtain a monetary estimate of a QALY. This chapter will also include first results of applying this approach in two different contexts. In one of the applications, we also extent this valuation to a broader well-being outcome measure, namely capability well-being, as extending the evaluative space of economic evaluations is of increasing importance and would also require a monetary valuation of the broader outcome measure. While the well-being valuation approach is not prone to framing biases like willingness to pay experiments, it comes with other caveats like the requirement of obtaining unbiased estimates of the well-being and impacts of income and health, which are notoriously difficult to obtain. Due to methodological differences and context dependency, it may, in general, never be possible to obtain one "true" estimate of the monetary value of a QALY in a society, but future research will further refine the ballpark in which this value may lie, which is informative for decision makers.

Keywords: value of health, QALY, capability approach, economic evaluation, life satisfaction approach

1 Introduction

"The monetary value of one year in full health is €30,000."

While such a statement seems at least controversial, if not offensive to many individuals, it relates to one of the key questions of the health economics discipline (Culyer and Maynard, 1997): What is the value of health? Asking and attempting to answering this question is not just a provocative thought experiment. It plays an important role in decision making for allocating scarce health care resources in many jurisdictions (Rowen *et al.*, 2017). Also outside of health economics and health care, a valuation of health and life can be pertinent to public policy making. Estimates of the monetary value of a statistical life are for example used for evaluating public policies relating to the environment and transportation safety (Ashenfelter, 2006).

A side note on the interpretation and context of a statement such as the one above: Initially, there may be moral objections to putting a monetary value on health (and therefore life) based on the notion that health is a special good, or a human right, whose value is immeasurable or infinite. Following this notion, health and health care, therefore, should not and cannot be traded-off between population groups or public sectors as the decision rule would be to maximise health no matter the costs. However, it seems that the democratic consensus is that we are not willing to invest all available resources in health care (increasing population health and survival), but also want to invest in other goods such as education, transportation or private consumption. That we do trade-off health to other goods has rarely been as obvious as during the current COVID-19 outbreak, where economic considerations of lockdown measures are directly weighted against health and lives of citizens. While governments may still claim that they are not willing to trade of lives for a less severe economic downturn (e.g. Olaf Scholz, the German minister of finance[2]), they are in essence doing exactly that by gradually relaxing lockdown measures even though the pandemic is not over, accepting a certain number of infections and deaths. An ordinary example for "sacrificing" your own health and the health of others on a more individual level would be the motorised private transport. In Germany in 2019 alone, 300,200 individuals were injured and 3,059 died as a results of road accidents (Destatis, 2020). The numbers for public transportation are almost at zero. Admittedly, public transportation is not a valuable alternative for many individuals, but those, who do use their own car instead public transport (if available), do this with the knowledge that they are risking theirs and others' health for gains in time and comfort. On a societal level, there seems to be the consensus that injuries and fatalities do not warrant a much higher investment in means of public transportation. Therefore, given these trade-offs, it is apparent that the value of health and life is not infinite. A second objection to the statement above may be that the value of health is expressed in monetary terms. However, money is the smallest common denominator in our society and the value has to be expressed that way to be informative for policy making as it relates decisions on the allocation of public budgets and funds.

Using and expanding the rational and the technical application of health economic evaluations and concepts like the Quality Adjusted Life Year (QALY),[3] this chapter will in particular advance as follows: First, it will be argued why the use of cost-effectiveness analysis, in general, is ethically justifiable and why its decision rule requires the estimation of a monetary value of health. Second, this chapter will provide an overview of the previously used methodologies and the corresponding results of previous attempts to estimate a monetary value of a QALY. Third, an alternative approach will be presented and first results from two studies estimating the monetary value of a QALY based on the well-being valuation approach will be summarised. One of the studies also

---

[2]　https://www.faz.net/aktuell/wirtschaft/corona-kirse-scholz-gegen-lockerung-wegen-wirtschaft-16701835.html (accessed 2 December 2020).

[3]　These frameworks and concepts are summarised in the previous chapter by Mitchell.

provides a corresponding estimate for a year in full capability well-being.[4] Lastly, this chapter will be put into a broader context.

2   Ethics of cost-effectiveness and its decision rule

There is increasing pressure on health care budgets due to an ageing population and the development of new (expensive) treatment options. Drastically expanding health care budgets aiming to provide all possible treatment options to everyone at any time does not seem to be a realistic way forward as outlined above. This raises the question, how decision-makers can decide on whether to reimburse certain health care services (or products) or not. Among many jurisdictions this assessment is operationalised using cost-effectiveness analysis (Rowen *et al.*, 2017), where the incremental costs of a new technology are compared to the expected incremental health gain it generates, which is measured using Quality Adjusted Life Years (QALYs) (Neumann *et al.*, 2016). On a side note, the QALY framework operates based on a certain understanding of health and disease, which in turn implies certain assumptions about the idea of the value of a medical interventions.[5] Furthermore important to note here, is that in countries like Germany or France, cost-effectiveness analysis and the QALY framework are not used in health technology assessment. The reasoning behind rejecting this approach more or less relate to either measurement concerns or moral objections. The following will touch on both aspects.

Coming back to the cost per QALY framework: Comparing health outcomes to costs of a treatment, may ultimately lead to some treatments not being available for certain patients based on partly monetary considerations. There are two aspects, which may be worth highlighting here, which, among other ethical considerations, were first (and likely better) formulated by Williams in the early days of QALYs and cost-effectiveness analysis (Williams, 1992; Williams, 1996):

First, economic evaluations support *collective*-priority setting in health care. This means that they are used on a health care level, somewhat detached from the clinical level without specific knowledge, who the patients are that are affected by certain decisions. While this is not exactly a 'veil of ignorance' as described by Rawls (Rawls, 1972), this detachment is the best option for allowing interpersonal judgements of life's value, which priority setting essentially is.

Second, when speaking of costs of a treatment and accepting that health care resources are limited, costs should be seen as 'what will have to be sacri-

---

[4]   This is also related to the concepts defined in the chapter by Mitchell.
[5]   The chapter by Stutzin Donoso discusses in detail that there competing interpretations are possible.

ficed' and especially what sacrifices have to be imposed on others. Every Euro spent on a certain treatment for one patient, may have been put to better use for another patient, whose health gains are now not realised. Williams (1992) considers disregarding costs in treatment decisions, meaning ignoring the sacrifices and subsequent adverse consequences imposed on others, as unethical. The use of QALYs as outcome measures is also not without limitations and includes several ethical concerns, which will not be discussed here, but are discussed in detail for example by Williams (1996) or Pinkerton et al. (2002).

If one accepts the notion that costs and effects of interventions have to be compared, the need for a monetary value for health can be derived from its decision rule. Equation (1) formulates the corresponding decision rule, with ΔE denoting the health gain (in QALYs) and ΔC the total costs compared to the alternative treatment:

$$\frac{\Delta C}{\Delta E} < v_Q \tag{1}$$

Taking a societal perspective, like is used in the Netherlands, this ratio, also called incremental cost-effectiveness ratio (ICER), is acceptable if it lies below the consumption value of a QALY v_Q, the so called threshold value, which would lead to a positive reimbursement decision for the health technology (Brouwer et al., 2019). The consumption value of health v_Q is the monetary value society attaches to one year in full health. In the Netherlands, v_Q is dependent on disease severity and the adaptive threshold value ranges from €20,000 to €80,000 per QALY. In the UK, the threshold value v_Q relates to the marginal cost-effectiveness of current spending in the health care system and was set to £20,000–30,000 per QALY (Claxton et al., 2011).

Without estimates or values for v_Q, the results of cost-effectiveness analyses are considerably less informative. Although it would still be possible to compare the ICERs of different interventions and assess which is more cost-effective, one could not assess whether the ICER of a certain intervention is still acceptable. Are costs of €100,000 per QALY for a certain intervention too much? Where should the line be drawn, if one accepts that health care budgets are limited and the value of health is not infinite? Explicit threshold values have not been formulated in many countries, and some countries, like Germany, even completely reject the cost-effectiveness framework altogether (Rowen et al., 2017). However, one needs to be aware of that even then, every decision on reimbursing (or not reimbursing) a certain health intervention to a certain price, implicitly produces a cost per QALY ratio for the specific intervention and disease area. Whether formulating and using an explicit threshold value leads to more efficient reimbursement decisions is not clear (yet), however such a system wide threshold would allow for a more transparent decision making.

3 Previous approaches for estimating the monetary value of a QALY

If and on what basis the threshold value v_Q, i.e. the value of health, is defined and used in health technology assessment varies widely across jurisdictions (Cameron *et al.*, 2018, Cleemput *et al.*, 2011). Due to its implications and importance, any such threshold value should have a strong empirical basis, which oftentimes may not be the case (Cameron *et al.*, 2018). A common challenge is that obtaining valid and informative estimates of v_Q is inherently difficult. There are currently two distinctly different types of methods based on demand sided approaches and supply sided approaches.

The latter approach entails estimating v_Q based on current health care spending and more specifically the marginal (health) returns to health spending. This value is often referred to as k-threshold (Brouwer *et al.*, 2019). The conceptual idea of the approach is the following: Given fixed health care budgets, the introduction of new health technologies is assumed to displace other existing treatments. The cost of implementing the new technology is then equal to the health foregone due to the displacement, i.e. the health opportunity cost. The threshold then represents the point at which more health is forgone than gained and is calculated as the average cost-effectiveness of all technologies and services that are displaced based on health spending data linked to health outcomes (van Baal *et al.*, 2019). In the first application of this approach, the k-threshold for the UK was estimated to be £12,936 per QALY (Claxton *et al.*, 2015). Similar studies have been conducted in Spain, with k-values of around €25,000 per QALY (Vallejo-Torres *et al.*, 2018), the Netherlands, with a base case estimate of €41,000 per QALY (van Baal *et al.*, 2019), and most recently in Sweden, where the marginal cost per life year was estimated to be €39,000 (Siverskog and Henriksson, 2019). While these kind of estimates are not affected by the shortcomings of stated preferences approaches and provide conceptually different valuations of a QALY, they do have limitations of their own. These mainly relate to the availability of suitable data (both on health care spending and outcomes) and the issues related to obtaining unbiased estimates of the effect of health care spending on mortality/morbidity. This type of approach is also most relevant in countries, which orient the threshold value on opportunity costs.

Demand sided approaches to estimating v_Q have a strong connection to welfare economics, as they relate to the societal willingness to pay (WTP) for a QALY. The cost per utility (QALY) of an intervention and this societal WTP then give a direct indication of the welfare impact of a health technology (Ryen and Svensson, 2015). There are two main empirical conceptualisations of obtaining this societal WTP: First, the value of a statistical life approach, which calculates the monetary value of preventing fatalities and is also used for evaluating public policies relating to the environment and transportation safety (Ashenfelter, 2006). This approach entails estimating the marginal rate of substitution between some welfare variable (wealth, income) and mortality risks either using stated preferences (hypothetical market situation) or revealed preferences methods (actual market behaviour). In a second step the value of a statistical life is converted to v_Q by relating this to the expected remaining life expectancy and quality of life with discounting future streams (Hirth et al., 2000). There are large methodological differences between studies, and the corresponding range of v_Q goes from €21,815 to €1,204,963 per QALY according to the review by Ryen et al. (2015), which included three such studies with 41 estimates. In a study that used a single estimate of the value of a statistical life for the UK (Mason et al., 2009), v_Q was estimated between €32,319 and €94,606. The drawback of the value of a statistical life approach is evident by these ranges: There are large degrees of freedom on how to estimate the value of a statistical life and on how to convert this to v_Q. It is therefore difficult to assess, which estimates should be used to inform the cost-effectiveness threshold.

A second demand sided approach, which is more commonly applied, is to ask representative samples directly about their WTP for incremental health or QALY gains using surveys and then aggregate these estimates to the WTP of a full QALY. While this was also done using discrete choice experiments (Gyrd-Hansen, 2003; van de Wetering et al., 2015), willingness to pay contingent valuation methods were predominantly used (Nimdet et al., 2015). These entailed for example describing two different health states (e.g. using EQ-5D profiles) and asking about how much individuals would be willing to pay for avoiding to be in the worse state. As the reviews by Ryen et al. (2015) and Nimdet et al. (2015) showed, there are however considerable differences in the design of such studies: Firstly, this relates to more conceptual differences as an individual or societal perspective (including altruistic motives), the type of population, whether to include only quality of life or also life expectancy, or whether scenarios were disease specific or about changes in general health (Ryen and Svensson, 2015). Secondly, there are various different types of elicitation procedures, like open-ended questions, bidding games, payment cart designs, dichotomous choice, or a combination thereof (Nimdet et al., 2015). This flexibility in designing such studies can be considered as a strength as it allows researchers to customise the design, control for certain influences, and adopt it to different contexts. However, this is also one of the reasons why estimates of v_Q vary widely across studies. Ryen et al. (2015) found a range across 24 articles going from less than €1,000 to €4,800,000 with trimmed mean and median estimates of €74,159 and €24,226 (in 2010 price levels) for one QALY. Another reason for finding such differences is that the framing of these questions and type of elicitation format plays an important role for the WTP results, which was specifically shown for example by Gyrd-Hansen et al. (2014) or Ahlert et al. (2016). This relates to the more general limitations of such stated preferences approaches, which lie in hypothetical response bias, insensitivity to scope or framing effects (Kling *et al.*, 2012).

4 The well-being valuation approach

A third and most recently developed demand sided approach for estimating v_Q is the so called well-being valuation approach, which has so far only been applied once in a study by Huang *et al.* (2018), and will be discussed in detail in this chapter. In this first application, v_Q for Australia was estimated to be between A\$42,000–A\$67,000 per QALY. In contrast to willingness-to-pay experiments, the well-being valuation approach does not directly ask individuals for a willingness to pay for a certain health gain, but relies on regression analysis and the well-being impacts of health and income to obtain a societal valuation of health. More specifically, the well-being valuation approach uses observational data to assess the experienced average impact of a change in a good on individuals' overall utility u, proxied by subjective well-being (SWB) or life satisfaction, and calculating the change in income necessary to maintain the same level of utility (Dolan and Fujiwara, 2016). This obtained monetary valuation is also known as compensating income variation (CV). To paraphrase, CV is the hypothetical, average amount of money you would need to give an individual so that he or she would be equally happy after imposing a certain change in his or her circumstances. In the following, this change in circumstances is a certain hypothetical change in health.

Therefore, while based on individual survey data, this approach is not a stated preferences approach, but also not a classical revealed preferences approach, as it does not involve actual market behaviour (Dolan and Fujiwara, 2016). The following will outline the conceptual model used for 1) estimating v_Q and an equivalent value for a year in full capability based on UK data and 2) estimating v_Q using large scale panel data from Germany. To quickly recap, the ICECAP-A would extend the evaluative space of health economic evaluations to capability well-being instead of a sole focus on health.[6] If this evaluative space is extended, it is important also to obtain estimates of the monetary value of a year in full capability (equivalent to v_Q) to be able to assess whether a certain interventions is cost-effective or not.

Applying the well-being valuation approach for estimating monetary values of capability well-being and health requires the following assumption about the relationship between health, capability and SWB: Individual's overall utility u, as proxied by SWB or life satisfaction (w), is a function of health or capability well-being h. This assumption is in conflict with how some see the

---

[6] Capability well-being, its potential role in health economic evaluations and its measurement via the ICECAP-A is described in the previous chapter by Mitchell.

relationship between capability, utility and SWB (Veenhoven, 2010), but it is a necessary assumption due to the mechanics of the well-being valuation approach. The conceptual model of the well-being valuation approach can be summarised as follows (this model was previously described by Ólafsdóttir et al., 2020):

$$u(h, y, x) = SWB(h, y, x) \tag{2}$$

Utility u is determined by health or capability well-being h, income y, and certain individual and socioeconomic characteristics summarised in vector x. An imposed health deterioration from h1 to h0 results in the utility decrement Δu:

$$\Delta u = u(y, h^0|x) - u(y, h^1|y) \tag{3}$$

The marginal rate of substitution or compensating income variation (CV) is the size of the change in income y necessary to equalise u before and after the health deterioration.

$$u(y + CV|h^0, x) = u(y|h^i, x) \tag{4}$$

Empirically, CV is estimated in two steps. First, the impact of income and health on SWB (or u) is calculated using regression analysis, controlling for demographics and possible confounders. Second, the coefficient estimates, which represent the marginal effects of income and health on SWB, are then divided by each other to obtain the marginal rate of substitution (or compensating variation) of income and health.

While the well-being valuation approach avoids some challenges associated with stated preferences methods, the use of observational data limits the scope to respondents' ex-post valuations with for example no means for explicitly including a societal perspective. Furthermore, endogeneity concerns are a prevailing issue of this approach as it relies on the estimation of causal effects of health and income to calculate their marginal trade-offs. While some of these concerns can be addressed, this has to be acknowledged when interpreting the results.

5   Applications of the well-being valuation approach

The following will summarise approaches and preliminary results for estimating v_Q based on the well-being valuation approach in two different context and based on two different types of data.

5.1 The value of a QALY and a year in full capability in the UK

In this case study, we estimated v_Q if its scope is limited to health and if it is extended to broader capability well-being (v_C) as measured through the ICE-CAP-A (Al-Janabi et al., 2012). We applied the well-being valuation approach to calculate a first monetary value for capability well-being in comparison to health, derived by utility weighted ICECAP-A and EQ-5D-5L values (corresponding to h in the above outlined framework), respectively (Devlin et al., 2018; Flynn et al., 2015). Data on health or well-being state h, life satisfaction w, and a number of control variables x, was obtained through an online survey, which was administered to a representative sample of UK citizens aged 18 to 65 (N=1,512) in February 2018. To overcome the endogeneity of income, a well-known issue in the well-being valuation literature (see e.g. Howley (2017) or Huang et al. (2018)), we applied an instrumental variable regression. The estimated impact of health or capability well-being h (summed up to 1 QALY or 1 year in full capability) on life satisfaction, the utility proxy, was then used to obtain estimates of v_Q and v_C.

Using the instrumental variable specification and a commonly applied logarithmic specification of income, our base case estimate of v_Q was £30,786 per QALY. The corresponding value for v_C, a year in full capability, was £66,597. The v_Q estimates compared well to previous estimates for the UK based on the value of a statistical life and willingness to pay experiments (Baker et al., 2010; Mason et al., 2009), while also being relatively close to NICE's threshold value (Claxton et al., 2011).

This first application is not without limitations, which mainly relate to obtaining unbiased estimates of the impact of income on life satisfaction. However, this is especially challenging in this rather small, cross-sectional sample. Assuming that the relative magnitudes of v_Q and v_C are unaffected by this, this application showed that if one would extent the evaluative space from health to capability well-being, a differential, larger threshold should be used in economic evaluations using the ICECAP-A measure. A more conceptual concern of this analysis lies in applying a utility-based approach to a capability measure. Utility and capability represent different concepts of value and their relationship and potential integration is not straightforward and will be subject of future research.[7]

Across different model specifications, the value of v_C was between 1.7 to 2.6 times larger than v_Q. A larger value could have been expected as capability well-being is broader (and more closely related to overall experienced utility) than merely health, but has not been empirically shown before. In a patient setting, capability well-being may capture care-related as well as medical or

---

[7]   This was also pointed out in the previous chapters by Mitchell and Ubels in this publication.

functional needs, while health as measured by the EQ-5D would be somewhat limited to the latter. This broader scope of capability instruments, covering both cure and care-related dimensions, was one of the rationales behind their development.[8] Hence, they might in particular be useful for a value-based assessment of settings with a broader understanding of cure and in particular care (e.g. long-term care, social care), where recipients represent rather clients than patients.

5.2 The value of a QALY in Germany

In this second application, we started out with the aim of estimating v_Q for Germany, as so far only one study provided such estimates based on willingness to pay experiments (Ahlert *et al.*, 2016). Their study was aptly called "How you ask is what you get [...]" referring the range of v_Q estimates they obtained from different contingent valuation designs (€3,911 to €43,115). The approach we used was similar to the one used by Huang *et al.* (2018) as we based our estimation on large-scale panel data. For this analysis, we used data from the German Socio-Economic Panel (SOEP) from 2002 to 2018 containing a final analysis sample of 29,735 individuals followed over multiple periods. The panel structure allowed us to run fixed effects regressions, removing the potential bias due to time-invariant unobservables. To further attempt to obtain unbiased estimates of the impact of income on life satisfaction, we applied an instrumental variable approach based on the industry-wage structure (Luechinger, 2009). The richness of the data furthermore allowed us to explore several empirical issues in applying the well-being valuation approach to valuing QALYs. This especially includes different functional form assumption of income (logarithmic, multiple income splines) or the or the health state dependence of the marginal utility of consumption (Finkelstein *et al.*, 2013).

The baseline fixed effects and instrumental variable regressions provided v_Q estimates of €58,533 and €22,717 per QALY for Germany. Estimated values varied across model specifications with the bulk of estimates lying between €20,000 and €60,000 and most instrumental variable estimates remaining rather stable around €20,000 per QALY. These estimates are somewhat larger compared to what has been found by Ahlert *et al.* (2016). Our study, which will be published in due course, furthermore adds to methodological and empirical challenges of applying the well-being valuation approach, in general, and for estimating the monetary value of a QALY in particular. Important to note here is that our estimates will not directly be relevant to health care decision making in Germany, as cost-effectiveness analysis is currently not used. While the

---

[8]   This is also discussed in the chapter by Mitchell.

arguments against using this framework – measurement issues or moral objections of e.g. putting a monetary value on health – are valid concerns, it needs to be acknowledged that the currently applied process has certain undesirable characteristics on its own: In Germany, new health technologies are only compared within an indication set (a certain disease) with no explicit comparison of costs and benefits. This process, for once, could lead to the situation that society (unknowingly) is paying a lot more for the same benefit in one disease compared to another disease. Within a cost-effectiveness framework, this differential weighting is more explicit (e.g. using a disease severity adaptive threshold like in the Netherlands) (Brouwer *et al.*, 2019).

6 Concluding remarks

This chapter attempted to illustrate (1) the ethics and decision rule of cost-effectiveness analysis (2) the subsequent need for obtaining monetary valuations of health if the principles of cost-effectiveness are accepted (3) how such values were previously estimated, and (4) presented a novel approach and first results from two studies also including monetary estimates of years in full capability well-being.

Coming back to the statement from the beginning of this chapter: While it should now be clear to readers, why such a value is needed and how it can be obtained, the following needs to be acknowledged: Although obtaining one "true" monetary value for a QALY in a society would be desirable (e.g. the €30,000 per QALY) as it would be most informative for decisions makers, obtaining such a value is not feasible. As becomes apparent from sections 3 and 4, estimates do not only differ considerably between conceptually different approaches, but also within the approaches themselves. The novel approach that was outlined and applied, is also not without limitations, but adds to this insofar as it further confirms and refines the *ballpark* of v_Q estimates from an individual perspective of between €20,000 and €60,000 for Germany and of around €30,000–40,000 per QALY for the UK. Future research into the application of the well-being valuation approach, willingness to pay experiments and the marginal returns of health spending to obtain monetary values of a QALY, will be valuable to further refine this ballpark. Another interesting observation from this chapter is that monetary estimates of a QALY based on opportunity costs (k-threshold) seem to be lower than estimates based on the societal value of a QALY. This implies that the health care budget is not set optimally and that there is underinvestment in health care (Brouwer *et al.*, 2019).

Independent of jurisdiction, given the ageing of western societies, the threats of global outbreaks, and, most importantly, the explosion of what is and will be medically possible in the near future, an efficient, equitable and transparent allocation of health care resources will be crucial. The cost-effectiveness framework and its decision rule based on what society is willing to pay or what has to be given up for certain health gains, or likely increasingly, certain well-being gains, can be one important tool to aid in achieving this. If countries like Germany will also make use of this tool in the future remains to be seen.[9] As a last remark, results from health economic evaluations rightfully are not, and likely never will be, the only basis on which decisions about which interventions should be made available to what patients will be based on. It merely represents the health economic perspective. Other ethical, medical, sociological or practical considerations should always play a role as well.

Acknowledgements: S. F. W. Himmler receives funding from the European Research Council (ERC) under the European Union's Horizon 2020 research and innovation programme (grant agreement No. 721402). The 2018 data collection was part of the COMPARE project and funded by the European Commission under the Horizon 2020 research and innovation programme (grant agreement No. 643476).

References

Ahlert, M., Breyer, F. and Schwettmann, L. (2016), "How you ask is what you get: Framing effects in willingness-to-pay for a QALY", *Social Science & Medicine*, Vol. 150, pp. 40–48.

Al-Janabi, H., N Flynn, T. and Coast, J. (2012), "Development of a self-report measure of capability wellbeing for adults: the ICECAP-A", *Quality of Life Research*, Vol. 21 No. 1, pp. 167–176.

Ashenfelter, O. (2006), "Measuring the Value of a Statistical Life: Problems and Prospects", *The Economic Journal*, Vol. 116 No. 510, pp. C10–C23.

van Baal, P., Perry-Duxbury, M., Bakx, P., Versteegh, M., van Doorslaer, E. and Brouwer, W. (2019), "A cost-effectiveness threshold based on the marginal returns of cardiovascular hospital spending", *Health Economics (United Kingdom)*, Vol. 28 No. 1, pp. 87–100.

Baker, R., Bateman, I., Donaldson, C., Jones-Lee, M., Lancsar, E., Loomes, G., Mason, H., Odejar, M., Pinto Prades, J. L., Robinson, A., Ryan, M., Shackley, P., Smith, R., Sugden, R. and Wildman, J. (2010), "Weighting and valuing quality-adjusted life-years using stated preference methods: Preliminary results from the social value of a QALY project", *Health Technology Assessment*, Vol. 14 No. 27.

Brouwer, W., van Baal, P., van Exel, J. and Versteegh, M. (2019), "When is it too expensive? Cost-effectiveness thresholds and health care decision-making", *European Journal of Health Economics*, Vol. 20 No. 2, pp. 175–180.

Cameron, D., Ubels, J. and Norström, F. (2018), "On what basis are medical cost-effectiveness thresholds set? Clashing opinions and an absence of data: a systematic review", *Global Health Action*, Vol. 11 No. 1.

---

[9] As is highlighted in the chapter by Buch *et al.*, other tools could relate to creating innovative reimbursement schemes for medical interventions.

Claxton, K., Martin, S., Soares, M., Rice, N., Spackman, E., Hinde, S., Devlin, N., Smith, P. C. and Sculpher, M. (2015), "Methods for the estimation of the National Institute for Health and care excellence cost-effectiveness threshold", *Health Technology Assessment*, Vol. 19 No. 14, pp. 1–503.

Claxton, K., Paulden, M., Gravelle, H., Brouwer, W. and Culyer, A. J. (2011), "Discounting and decision making in the economic evaluation of health-care technologies", *Health Economics*, Vol. 20 No. 1, pp. 2–15.

Cleemput, I., Neyt, M., Thiry, N., De Laet, C. and Leys, M. (2011), "Using threshold values for cost per quality-adjusted life-year gained in healthcare decisions", *International Journal of Technology Assessment in Health Care*, Vol. 27 No. 1, pp. 71–76.

Culyer, T. and Maynard, A. K. eds. (1997), Being Reasonable about the Economics of Health: Selected Essays by Alan Williams, In Edward Elgar: Cheltenham.

Destatis (2020), Pressemitteilung Nr. 061 vom 27. Februar 2020, available from: https://www.destatis.de/DE/Presse/Pressemitteilungen/2020/02/PD20_061_46241.html (accessed 2 December 2020).

Devlin, N. J., Shah, K. K., Feng, Y., Mulhern, B. and van Hout, B. (2018), "Valuing health-related quality of life: An EQ-5D-5L value set for England", *Health Economics (United Kingdom)*, Vol. 27 No. 1, pp. 7–22.

Dolan, P. and Fujiwara, D. (2016), Happiness-Based Policy Analysis, In *The Oxford Handbook of Well-Being and Public Policy*, chapter 10, Adler MD, Fleurbaey M (eds). Oxford University Press; 1–41.

Finkelstein, A., Luttmer, E. F. P. and Notowidigdo, M. J. (2013), "What good is health without wealth? The effect of health on the marginal utility of consumption", *Journal of the European Economic Association*, Vol. 11, pp. 221–258.

Flynn, T. N., Huynh, E., Peters, T. J., Al-Janabi, H., Clemens, S., Moody, A. and Coast, J. (2015), "Scoring the ICECAP-A capability instrument. Estimation of a UK general population tariff", *Health Economics (United Kingdom)*, Vol. 24 No. 3, pp. 258–269.

Gyrd-Hansen, D. (2003), "Willingness to pay for a QALY", *Health Economics*, Vol. 12 No. 12, pp. 1049–1060.

Gyrd-Hansen, D., Jensen, M. L. and Kjaer, T. (2014), "Framing the willingness-to-pay question: Impact on response pattern and mean willingness to pay", *Health Economics*, Vol. 23 No. 5, pp. 550–563.

Hirth, R. A., Chernew, M. E., Miller, E., Fendrick, A. M. and Weissert, W. G. (2000), "Willingness to Pay for a Quality-adjusted Life Year: In Search of a Standard", *Medical Decision Making*, Vol. 20 No. 3, pp. 332–342.

Howley, P. (2017), "Less money or better health? Evaluating individual's willingness to make trade-offs using life satisfaction data", *Journal of Economic Behavior and Organization*, Vol. 135, pp. 53–65.

Huang, L., Frijters, P., Dalziel, K. and Clarke, P. (2018), "Life satisfaction , QALYs , and the monetary value of health", *Social Science & Medicine*, Vol. 211 No. June, pp. 131–136.

Kling, C. L., Phaneuf, D. J. and Zhao, J. (2012), "From Exxon to BP: Has Some Number Become Better than No Number?", *Journal of Economic Perspectives*, Vol. 26 No. 4, pp. 3–26.

Luechinger, S. (2009), "Valuing Air Quality Using the Life Satisfaction Approach", *The Economic Journal*, Vol. 119, pp. 482–515.

Mason, H., Jones-Lee, M. and Donaldson, C. (2009), "Modelling the monetary value of a QALY: a new approach based on UK data", *Health Economics*, Vol. 18 No. 8, pp. 933–950.

Neumann, P. J., Sanders, G. D., Russell, L. B., Siegel, J. E. and Ganiats, T. G. (2016), *Cost Effectiveness in Health and Medicine*. Oxford University Press: New York.

Nimdet, K., Chaiyakunapruk, N., Vichansavakul, K. and Ngorsuraches, S. (2015), "A systematic review of studies eliciting willingness-to-pay per quality-adjusted life year: Does it justify ce threshold?", *PLoS ONE*, Vol. 10 No. 4, pp. 1–16.

Ólafsdóttir, T., Ásgeirsdóttir, T. L. and Norton, E. C. (2020), "Valuing pain using the subjective well-being method", *Economics and Human Biology*, Vol. 37.

Pinkerton, S. D., Johnson-Masotti, A. P., Derse, A. and Layde, P. M. (2002), "Ethical issues in cost-effectiveness analysis", *Evaluation and Program Planning*, Vol. 25 No. 1, pp. 71–83.

Rawls, J. (1972), *A Theory of Justice*. Oxford University Press.

Rowen, D., Azzabi Zouraq, I., Chevrou-Severac, H. and van Hout, B. (2017), "International Regulations and Recommendations for Utility Data for Health Technology Assessment", *PharmacoEconomics*, Vol. 35 No. s1, pp. 11–19.

Ryen, L. and Svensson, M. (2015), "The Willingness to Pay for a Quality Adjusted Life Year: A Review of the Empirical Literature", *Health Economics*, Vol. 24 No. 10, pp. 1289–1301.

Siverskog, J. and Henriksson, M. (2019), "Estimating the marginal cost of a life year in Sweden's public healthcare sector", *The European Journal of Health Economics*, Vol. 20 No. 5, pp. 751–762.

Vallejo-Torres, L., García-Lorenzo, B. and Serrano-Aguilar, P. (2018), "Estimating a cost-effectiveness threshold for the Spanish NHS", *Health Economics (United Kingdom)*, Vol. 27 No. 4, pp. 746–761.

Veenhoven, R. (2010), "Capability and happiness: Conceptual difference and reality links", *Journal of Socio-Economics*, Vol. 39 No. 3, pp. 344–350.

Wetering, L. van de, van Exel, J., Bobinac, A. and Brouwer, W. B. F. (2015), "Valuing QALYs in Relation to Equity Considerations Using a Discrete Choice Experiment", *PharmacoEconomics*, Vol. 33 No. 12, pp. 1289–1300.

Williams, A. (1992), "Cost-effectiveness analysis: is it ethical?", *Journal of Medical Ethics*, No. 18, pp. 7–11.

Williams, A. (1996), "Qalys and ethics: A health economist's perspective", *Social Science and Medicine*, Vol. 43 No. 12, pp. 1795–1804.

Risk-sharing schemes to finance expensive pharmaceuticals

Interdisciplinary analyses

Charlotte Buch / Jan Schildmann / Jürgen Zerth

Abstract

Limited resources for healthcare need to be allocated effectively and efficiently and in accordance with the respective value of medical interventions. Recent developments in the pharmaceutical market and a rise in the cost of drugs pose a challenge for healthcare systems. This is particularly the case for so-called "personalized medicine" and drugs for small numbers of patients (e.g. orphan drugs). Research and development costs are high, while there are risks in terms of financial return, given that these drugs only address a very small patient population. Challenges to assess the value of these drugs are considerable, especially considering the lack of robust data due to small clinical studies. Accordingly, there is a high uncertainty regarding the real-world effectiveness, leading to significant discrepancies between the pharmaceutical company's list price and the cost payer's willingness to pay.

One approach to control pharmaceutical expenditures in these cases is value-based pricing. On a microperspective level, this is employed as risk-sharing agreements between payers and pharmaceutical companies, whereby the uncertainties, i.e. risks, regarding the clinical and economic performance are shared and the remuneration for the drug is dependent on its real-world value. Depending on the inclusion of an outcome element into the scheme, we can distinguish financial-based risk-sharing schemes and performance- or outcome-based risk-sharing agreements.

This chapter will analyse the strengths and weaknesses of performance- or outcome-based risk-sharing agreements (PBRSA). In addition to a theoretical analysis, we will substantiate it by reference to a case study of a PBRSA involving the evaluation of drugs for a multiple sclerosis risk-sharing scheme in the United Kingdom.

Keywords: risk-sharing, pharmaceuticals, value-based pricing, performance-based risk-sharing agreements

1 Introduction

Some medical drugs come at an extraordinary price. One of the more recent examples is Onasemnogen Abeparvovec (Zolgensma®), a gene therapy for the neuromuscular disorder spinal muscular atrophy. It was approved by the United States Food and Drugs Administration in May 2019 and induces high costs considering direct drug treatment and non-treatment costs (Pearson *et al.*, 2019, p. 1302). Given that the drug was the most expensive medical therapy in the world at the time of approval, it attracted a lot of attention in discussions by experts and the public. However, the drug example named, which is supposed to be administered only once to the patient, represents only one side of higher expenditures for pharmaceuticals. There are other pharmaceuticals that induce high expenditures because of an enduring level of the prescription itself or changes in prescribed medications (e.g. substitutions from low-dose approaches to higher-dose ones) (Lohmüller *et al.*, 2019).

In Germany, the expenditures of the German Statutory Health Insurance for pharmaceuticals are close to those for outpatient care. This means that pharmaceuticals already belong to the most expensive service areas (GKV-Spitzenverband, 2019, p. 4; Pfannstiel *et al.*, 2019, p. 313). These expenditures have been increasing constantly over the last few years (GKV-Spitzenverband, 2019, p. 7). We have to differentiate two end-points of a continuum to specify potential reasons for higher expenditures, as has been already mentioned above. The increase of expenditures may be generated by (1) a rise in the number of units of drugs or (2) the proportion of drugs that can be connected with a higher price compared to permissible comparator therapy (Evaluate, 2019; Statistisches Bundesamt, 2019, p. 44). In this respect, new and possibly innovative pharmaceuticals are cost drivers because of two different reasons that may sometimes interact. First of all, higher expenditures may result from targeting a large number of patients that can be addressed by the medical innovation (population approach). Secondly, as it is the case with Onasemnogen Abeparvovec, a pharmaceutical solution has been developed for a very small population whereby pharmaceutical companies aim at recovering their higher development costs by employing price mark-ups.[1] Further examples are so-called orphan drugs, which are drugs for very rare diseases, and targeted drugs, which are used, for example, for cancer patients with a certain genetic mutation (Pfannstiel *et al.*, 2019, pp. 313–314).

Rising costs for medical drugs point to fundamental issues: The resources that are available within a healthcare system based on solidarity have to be restricted and limited. Consequently, there is an ongoing societal debate and

---

[1]   Differentiation of high-risk approaches from the population approach could be beneficial referring to traditional public health considerations Edwards and Atenstaedt (2019, p. 11).

consensus needed to find an appropriate match that citizens could claim having access to a certain level of healthcare and healthcare innovations, and, concomitantly, the additional financial burden for those citizens may only increase moderately.[2] At the same time and while considering the difficulties in stemming the rise of pharmaceutical expenditures, it is important to keep or build incentives for the development of new effective medical drugs. While there are limited data available on the costs of drug development (Morgan *et al.*, 2011, pp. 10–11), it seems fair to assume that the research and development of new drugs in many cases needs large financial investments combined with a long and uncertain research and development process. This is especially the case for those fields of applications where only a small number of beneficiaries could be targeted, such as in the case of rare diseases and those with an unmet medical need, i.e. when there is a higher investment risk. Therefore, while payers are searching for cost-containment measures, it is also important to consider options to keep pharmaceutical companies encouraged to be innovative (Danzon, 2018; Pfannstiel *et al.*, 2019, p. 308). In the following, we provide a brief account of some of the price-regulations schemes used in different healthcare systems to reconcile the aforementioned interests of payers, the pharmaceutical industry, patients and other stakeholders.

2 Challenges of expensive pharmaceuticals – the impact of a risk-based regulation scheme

Referring to the challenges mentioned above, healthcare systems in industrialized countries have to find an appropriate trade-off between controlling expenditures within the regulated benefit basket and fostering innovation and ensuring access to new diagnosis and treatment options (Levaggi, 2014, p. 69).[3] Employing drug price regulation is one of the standard approaches employed to meet that optimisation problem and is directly connected with elaborating some forms of a value for money measurement. One specific strategy is based on so-called value-based pricing.

---

[2]   See the chapter by Stutzin Donoso in this publication for a general discussion of the concept of health and right to healthcare.

[3]   The chapter by Alex in this publication also deals with the question of sustainable healthcare.

2.1 Risk-sharing within a value-based regulation approach

Value-based pricing approaches are rooted within a legitimation of a price by its impact on a perceived or estimated value to the patient.[4] Different strategies of value-based pricing on the macroeconomic level have been implemented. An incremental cost effectiveness ratio is used, for example, to give an appraisal for developing a price cap for pharmaceutical reimbursement in the United Kingdom (UK), as a Beveridge-type country (OECD, 2010, p. 166). Bismarckian-type countries, such as Germany, believe in the idea that decentralized regulated competition is an additional means for elaborating "value for money", fostering variations in preference and willingness to pay. However, regardless of the macroeconomic approaches chosen by different countries, fostering the development of new drugs while bearing in mind limited resources is the definite optimisation problem which each healthcare system faces.

Against the background of rising costs for medical drugs and limits of established models for financing new drugs, we will focus in the following on risk-sharing agreements utilising value-based pricing which have been developed as one standardized approach to control pharmaceutical expenditures.

Risk-sharing agreements can be defined as

> agreements concluded by payers and pharmaceutical companies to diminish the impact on the payer's budget of new and existing medicines brought about by either the uncertainty of the value of the medicine and/or the need to work within finite budgets. (Adamski *et al.*, 2010)

According to the logic of risk-sharing agreements, pharmaceutical companies grant some kind of warranty for the value of a medical drug. The company and the payer both have different obligations depending on the occurrence of an agreed condition (Adamski *et al.*, 2010; Renze-Westendorf, 2010, p. 206).

Participants of risk-sharing agreements acknowledge that there are uncertainties regarding developing and marketing a medical drug, i.e. risks regarding the clinical and economic performance in the real world. It is not clear whether the effectiveness of a medical drug in clinical reality, particularly at the time of its admission, reflects the efficacy shown in clinical trials (Antonanzas *et al.*, 2011, p. 399, 2011, p. 399; Garrison *et al.*, 2013, p. 704). These uncertainties are especially considerable for new, innovative and expensive drugs that only address small target populations. The reason for this is that clinical studies are small in such cases and, therefore, the accompanying evidence is sparse. Accordingly, there is an outcome uncertainty in terms of the

---

[4]   Further discussions on different judgements of value from healthcare interventions can be read in Vermeulen and Krabbe (2018). See the chapter by Steigenberger *et al.* in this publication for information about how to integrate the patients' perspective into the value assessment of medical interventions.

patients' response to treatment and how that will translate into health outcomes and resource utilisation, as well as a subgroup uncertainty, i.e. which patients of the heterogeneous population should and do get treated (Carlson et al., 2010, p. 188).

From the payer's point of view, these uncertainties are even more pronounced by the inherent characteristic of drugs as a post-launch "experience" good. Consequently, there is a specific risk of an ongoing asymmetry of information between the pharmaceutical company and different cost-payers considering the results of the implementation of the new drug, especially the number of prescriptions by doctors and the valuation of the beneficiaries. Controlling the expected profit margin in these cases is very complex for the pharmaceutical company from an *ex ante* perspective. If payers are additionally risk-averse, i.e. they have a greater fear of incorrectly paying than not paying for a cost-ineffective technology, they will insist on paying only for the (most) effective healthcare interventions within their limited budget (Towse and Garrison, 2010, p. 94).

Considering that assumption, pharmaceutical companies run the risk that the real-world value of a manufactured drug is underestimated. In the worst case, the payer refuses to adopt the drug at all (Garrison et al., 2013, p. 704). In addition, there may be high development costs and manufacturing overheads for a potentially curative or, at least, disease-modifying therapy that is only applicable to a small market and must be compensated by high list prices (Editorial, 2019, p. 697).

Pharmaceutical companies and cost-payers have different priorities regarding the payment because they have different information and views about the value of a new drug and the allocation of the accompanying risks. However, one potential shared interest is an objective assessment of benefits and costs. Obviously, such a value-oriented assessment is especially important for very expensive pharmaceuticals because there is a lot at stake for both sides: The pharmaceutical company wants its expenses for research and development to be compensated, while the payer needs to weigh the new drug against other therapies they may no longer be able to fund. In particular cases in which evidence is limited at the time of admission of the drug, for example, due to small studies for an orphan disease, it may be possible that the payer and manufacturer cannot align their expectations of remuneration and the company decides to drop out rather than to accept the price of the payer.

In order to avoid this situation, risk-sharing schemes enable the risk mentioned to be shared between payer and manufacturer by making the value of the drug, i.e. the price or remuneration, dependent on the value of the product, i.e. the future proven effectiveness in the real world (OECD, 2010, p. 170). Hereby, the payments to be made will be fixed *ex ante* and are contingent on information that will be collected *ex post* (Antonanzas et al., 2011, p. 400). Such value-based schemes may not only help to control pharmaceutical expenditures without negatively impacting the patient populations but also enable discounts without changing the high list price. This is relevant from the perspective of the pharmaceutical company, because the list price serves as an international comparison and changes may affect manufacturers' global revenues (Carlson *et al.*, 2010, p. 188; Towse and Garrison, 2010, pp. 95–96).

Risk-sharing agreements can be distinguished according to either financial/financial-based schemes or outcome/performance-based models (Adamski *et al.*, 2010).

2.2 Financial-based risk-sharing agreements

Finance-based schemes do not usually take the patient outcome into account but concentrate more on keeping the expenditures within agreed limits (Adamski *et al.*, 2010). Some examples of this risk-sharing approach are price volume agreements or budget impact schemes, according to which the unit price of a product is linked to the volumes sold. An increase of the volume of units results in a declining cost per unit. This is especially important when there is a possibility that the new medicine will be prescribed in a wider population than anticipated (Adamski *et al.*, 2010; OECD, 2010, p. 170).

Another form of financial-based risk-sharing is patient access schemes, which seek to enhance the value of new drugs and improve the possibility of their funding. They involve either the use of a drug for free or with financial discounts for an agreed period of time, or they focus on controlling the financial impact from an individual patient's perspective in the form of price capping schemes. The latter are connected to a specific outcome element, for example, when the drugs are provided for free once patients have exceeded a specified number of units but need more to support a certain state of health. Such an arrangement prevents the payer from spending more than a fixed amount per patient (Adamski *et al.*, 2010; OECD, 2010, p. 171).

2.3 Performance-based risk-sharing agreements

Performance-based risk-sharing schemes – also called performance-based-risk sharing agreements (PBRSA) – address the optimisation of definite healthcare expenditures as well. However, different from financed-based models, these schemes are dependent on the generation of evidence regarding the real-world impact of a given drug on patients' health. The remuneration depends on the (real-world) effectiveness of the drug according to data collection subsequent to the admission of the drug. Remuneration is determined either directly by a pre-arranged rule or indirectly through an agreement regarding the option to renegotiate prices if a certain condition has been met (Adamski *et al.*, 2010; Garrison *et al.*, 2013, p. 705). The outcomes, which serve as a basis for the remuneration, may be defined either in terms of outcome-related benefits (e.g. clinical response) or cost-effectiveness (e.g. cost per quality-adjusted life year[5]), each at the individual patient level or the aggregated level of the whole population treated (OECD, 2010, p. 172).

There are different types of PBRSA: Using outcome guarantees, the treatment costs for patients not reaching a predetermined response are (fully or partially) paid back by the manufacturer. One prominent example which has been discussed in this regard is the coverage for CAR T-cells (Jørgensen *et al.*, 2020). Another type of PBRSA involves coverage with evidence development. This approach means that there is access to a new drug while evidence is generated within a given period of time. However, reimbursement may change during the course of this time depending on the findings regarding predetermined health outcomes. Finally, PBRSA involving conditional treatment continuation means that reimbursement only takes place if patients achieve a previously defined level of response (Gonçalves *et al.*, 2018).

Implementing a successful PBRSA needs some serious preliminary considerations. In particular, the costs of generating additional evidence or information on treatment response must be weighed against the benefits that better resource allocation decisions bring, which is basically an investment decision. All parties have to decide beforehand whether a PBRSA is acceptable to them in the given situation and with the given risk. In addition, there is the need for consideration regarding how the PBRSA should be implemented and evaluated to be successful. Among the many questions which must be answered are the choice of the appropriate study design and outcome parameters, consideration about who will measure these parameters and in which time frame, what the reimbursement modalities will look like and a lot more (Garrison *et al.*, 2013, p. 709). These questions are raised by different interests that have to be embedded within the PBRSA.

The PBRSA approach seems appropriate if there is a significant uncertainty regarding the effectiveness of a given drug, while, at the same time, there is the desire to provide patients with access to its potential benefit. Therefore, it is especially interesting for funding new and innovative medicines such as orphan drugs and gene therapies. In contrast to this, finance-based schemes are more useful for generics, where one assumes that the outcome is already known and does not need to be considered (Carlson *et al.*, 2010, p. 180; Gonçalves *et al.*, 2018).

---

[5] The cost-effectiveness approach is further discussed in the chapter by Himmler in this publication. See the chapters by Mitchell and Ubels in this publication for more information about quality-adjusted life years and their alternatives.

A second interesting feature of PBRSAs is that there is the possibility of generating additional evidence. The latter is a desirable public good since it is not only valuable regarding the certain drug to be assessed, but it also offers insights into the respective disease itself and, therefore, enables a general improvement of patient care.

Given the preceding analysis, PBRSAs seem potentially desirable from an ethical and societal perspective. However, it is necessary to analyse the advantages and barriers of a PBRASA to determine its value and possible limitations in practice (Garrison et al., 2013, pp. 717–718). The multiple sclerosis (MS) risk-sharing scheme, which has been established in the UK, is an illustrative example to learn about a PBRSA in practice and its associated strengths and weaknesses. This case example will be described and, subsequently, the benefits and problems with implementation of PBRSAs in practice will be discussed in the following.

3   Case example: The multiple sclerosis risk-sharing scheme in the UK

Treatment for the chronic disease relapsing-remitting MS was restricted to anti-inflammatory drugs, such as cortisone, and symptomatic treatment up until the mid-1990s. Treatment options changed when the first disease-modifying therapies, interferon beta and glatiramer acetate, were developed. While these drugs do not cure the disease, they at least reduce the number of relapses. Four different pharmaceutical companies had licensed respective products (three interferon beta products and one glatiramer) within a rather short time frame. The problem with those drugs from a payer perspective was that it was not possible to predict their long-term effect from their short-term clinical achievements shown in clinical studies. Therefore, the National Institute for Health and Wellbeing came to the conclusion in its initial assessment in 2002 that the disease-modifying therapies were not cost-effective and should not be funded by the National Health Service (NICE, 2002).

Several stakeholders were obviously disappointed by this decision and campaigned against it. One argument was that cost-effectiveness may be derived if the short-term successes could also be proven in the long-term. Therefore, the first risk-sharing scheme in the UK was established to examine the long-term development of and to enable patients' access to the therapies.

The subject of the scheme were the four MS drugs. The stakeholders involved were the respective pharmaceutical companies, the UK Department of Health and representatives of patients and health professionals. Around 5000 patients in 70 MS specialist centres across the UK were recruited in the scheme within three years. They were monitored over ten years by capturing their

Expended Disability Status Scale status every year. The natural development of the disease was projected as a comparator, based on data from a historic control group, to assess the impact of the therapies. Regarding reimbursement, the stakeholders agreed on a cost-effectiveness threshold of 36,000 £ per quality-adjusted life year, which had to be kept. Therefore, the pharmaceutical companies lowered the price of their products right at the beginning and agreed that the impact of the therapies would be analysed every two years. The health outcome (effect of the drug on the progression of disease) was determined for any drug evaluated. In the case of missing the predetermined target outcome, the price of the respective therapy would be further lowered (Department of Health, 2002, pp. 7–14).

According to this agreement, the long-term clinical and outcome impact and cost-effectiveness of the disease-modifying therapies were examined. Six years after the start of the scheme, the findings about the longer-term effectiveness of the drugs were still mixed (Palace et al., 2015, pp. 502–504), but the additional data gathered during the scheme showed that there was a clinically significant treatment effect maintained at 10 years, reducing the progression of the disease, decreasing over time. If this effect was maintained over 20 years, the cost-effectiveness target would be reached (Palace et al., 2019, pp. 257–259).

4 Discussion

The strengths and limitations to implement this approach to share the risks of new and costly drugs will be discussed in the following based on the example of the MS scheme and the preceding theoretical analyses.

4.1 Strengths of PBRSA (in the context of the MS risk-sharing scheme)

One of the positive experiences of the MS risk-sharing scheme was that it had a strong impact on the care of patients with MS in the UK in addition to the generation of evidence on the effectiveness and cost-effectiveness of the drugs involved. Most importantly, the MS specialist centres, which had been partially newly established at the time of the scheme, have now build a strong network improving the support of and care for MS patients in terms of quantity and quality. In addition, many new MS therapists, nurses and doctors have been trained and educated since this has also been part of the companies' obligations. It should be noted that many patients were getting access to the therapies due to the scheme which would otherwise not have been possible. In addition to the change of structural aspects relevant to the high quality of care for patients with MS, the data generated within the scheme over a long time period offers valuable insights into the disease itself for all stakeholders, such as its long-term development, and enables improved care (Boggild *et al.*, 2009).

Apart from these advantages shown in the real world, theory hints at even more benefits. First of all and relevant from the perspective of payers, they allow patients' access to innovative medicines and, therefore, to a broader range of treatment options and potential health benefits. Furthermore, pharmaceutical companies are encouraged to develop new drugs, which contribute to the health of those patient populations where health gain, hence value, is greatest. For the payers, the additional evidence generated in the course of a PRBSA decreases uncertainties about effectiveness and informs decisions about allocation within a limited budget. On the other hand, the pharmaceutical companies gain faster market access for their innovative medicines, because they can prove their real-world value over time. Since the terms of agreement between payer and manufacturer are usually confidential, this offers the possibility of hidden discounts and, therefore, remains neutral regard list prices, which are relevant for the global market. Another advantage is that PBRSAs allow the definition of patient groups which are likely to benefit from the treatment. Thereby, both manufacturers and payers reduce the risk of using the drug in patient groups not likely to profit from the new treatment (Adamski *et al.*, 2010; Gonçalves *et al.*, 2018).

4.2 Weaknesses (in the context of the MS risk-sharing scheme)

Given the possible strengths of PBRSAs, they seem an "understandable and logical response to increasing pressure for greater evidence of real-world effectiveness and long-term cost-effectiveness for new medicines" (Garrison *et al.*, 2013, p. 717). However, they do not come without disadvantages and barriers for implementation. Firstly and relevant for the pharmaceutical companies is that they have to show their hypotheses of the suggested treatment effect in a real-world environment, which means there is new risk of calculating their contribution margin. This perspective may already be sufficient to hinder the implementation of a PBRSA. Even if the parties agree in principle regarding a PBRSA, implementing and monitoring PBRSAs cause financial and administrative burdens. It is important to evaluate these investment costs against the potential benefits of PBRSAs and, of course, to find a fair solution regarding carrying the financial and administrative burden.

One challenge is the difficulty of defining appropriate performance indicators that are easily measurable and, at the same time, adequate to demonstrate effectiveness. Similar to clinical studies, there may be situations in which surrogate parameters may be easy to collect, whereas direct indicators to demonstrate effectiveness, such as overall survival in cancer care, are difficult to obtain – particularly in diseases with a longer course. An additional barrier for the payer may be an insufficient infrastructure for collecting, analysing and monitoring data. There may also be ethico-legal challenges concerning data protection and the need to find agreements for further proceedings after the agreement about a scheme ends (Adamski et al., 2010; Garrison et al., 2013, p. 718; Gonçalves et al., 2018; Lorente et al., 2019, p. 30; Neumann, 2013, p. 701).

Further problems and concerns can be identified regarding the case example of the MS risk-sharing scheme in the UK. One important point of criticism in this concrete example was that the historic control group did not represent the actual state-of-the-art regarding the treatment of MS prior to the start of the scheme. In addition, there were questions concerning the neglect of quality standards. Furthermore, measuring the impact of the treatments using only the Expended Disability Status Scale scores was shown to be difficult given the heterogeneity of the presentation of MS and the differing courses of progression. Additionally, many reasons led to the delay of evidence generation. The long observation period caused difficulties as well, for example, many administrative challenges. Last but not least, new medicines against MS were developed during the course of the scheme, therefore, when the final results of the scheme came out they had mostly already been outdated (Adamski et al., 2010; Boggild et al., 2009; Palace et al., 2019, pp. 258–259).

Nevertheless, it was possible to find remedies to some of these problems during the scheme, for example, by adapting the control group and the research methodology (Palace et al., 2015, pp. 502–504). Moreover, even with the development of new treatment approaches during the scheme, the results generated have important consequences for assessing the cost-effectiveness of present and future MS drugs (Palace et al., 2019, pp. 257–259).

5   Conclusion

The application of PBRSAs keeps promises as well as the risk of failing, as has been shown in theory and in the case study included (Antonanzas et al., 2011, p. 393). Correct planning seems one key to the successful implementation of PRBSAs. This includes detailed considerations regarding unambiguous and easily measured effectiveness criteria, transparency and ethical considerations, as well as staffing and funding considerations. The PBRSAs should only be considered when there are explicit and transparent objectives and scopes, when the new drug is a novel treatment in a high priority disease area with only a few or no effective alternative treatments, and when a likely health gain can be determined within a limited amount of time. Alternatively, PBRSAs should be rejected when effective and low-cost treatment standards already exist or when health authorities could end up funding a substantial part of the new drug's development costs. The high administrative burden must be weighed against the likely health and/or financial benefits. The patients' compliance must always be considered and addressed in the scheme proposed (Adamski *et al.*, 2010)[6].

At present, it is unclear whether and where PBRSAs can really be embedded within the beneficiaries' focus (Levaggi, 2014, p. 72; Neumann, 2013, p. 702). However, they may be become more prevalent in the future, given the fact that there is lack of robust evidence according to which it is possible to predict real-world effectiveness at the time of admission for many drugs in the times of "personalized" or "precision" medicine. The distinction here between Bismarckian- and Beveridge-type healthcare systems may become very interesting: Considering the baseline philosophy of Bismarckian-types, PBRSAs may be interpreted as an further attempt to use controlled selective contracting in order to collect appropriate information about value for money. Considering current discussions on converging national high technology assessment approaches and methods, PBRSAs could play an important role within a European method box.

References

Adamski, J., Godman, B., Ofierska-Sujkowska, G., Osińska, B., Herholz, H., Wendykowska, K., Laius, O., Jan, S., Sermet, C., Zara, C., Kalaba, M., Gustafsson, R., Garuolienè, K., Haycox, A., Garattini, S. and Gustafsson, L. L. (2010), "Risk sharing arrangements for pharmaceuticals: potential considerations and recommendations for European payers", *BMC health services research*, Vol. 10 No. 153.

Antonanzas, F., Juarez-Castello, C. and Rodriguez-Ibeas, R. (2011), "Should health authorities offer risk-sharing contracts to pharmaceutical firms? A theoretical approach", *Health economics, policy, and law*, Vol. 6 No. 3, pp. 391–403.

Boggild, M., Palace, J., Barton, P., Ben-Shlomo, Y., Bregenzer, T., Dobson, C. and Gray, R. (2009), "Multiple sclerosis risk sharing scheme: two year results of clinical cohort study with historical comparator", *BMJ*, Vol. 339, b4677.

Carlson, J. J., Sullivan, S. D., Garrison, L. P., Neumann, P. J. and Veenstra, D. L. (2010), "Linking payment to health outcomes: a taxonomy and examination of performance-based reimbursement schemes between healthcare payers and manufacturers", *Health policy*, Vol. 96 No. 3, pp. 179–190.

Danzon, P. M. (2018), "Differential Pricing of Pharmaceuticals: Theory, Evidence and Emerging Issues", *PharmacoEconomics*, Vol. 36 No. 12, pp. 1395–1405.

Department of Health (2002), *Cost effective provision of disease modifying therapies for people with Multiple Sclerosis, Health Service Circular.*

Editorial (2019), "Gene therapy's next installment", *Nature biotechnology*, Vol. 37 No. 7, p. 697.

---

[6]   How to increase the patient compliance by implementing shared decision-making is discussed in detail in the chapter by Napiwodzka in this publication.

Edwards, R. T. and Atenstaedt, R. (2019), "Introduction to public health und public health economics", in Edwards, R. T. and McIntosh, E. (Eds.), *Applied Health Economics for Public Health Practice and Research*, Oxford University Press, pp. 1–26.

Evaluate (2019), "Weltweiter Arzneimittelumsatz von verschreibungspflichtigen Generika und Originalpräparaten in den Jahren von 2006 bis 2024 (in Milliarden US-Dollar)", Cited by de.statista.com, available at: https://de.statista.com/statistik/daten/studie/311686/umfrage/weltweiter-arzneimittelumsatz-von-verschreibungspflichtigen-generika-und-originalpraeparaten/ (accessed 2 December 2020).

Garrison, L. P., Towse, A., Briggs, A., Pouvourville, G. de, Grueger, J., Mohr, P. E., Severens, J. L. H., Siviero, P. and Sleeper, M. (2013), "Performance-based risk-sharing arrangements-good practices for design, implementation, and evaluation. Report of the ISPOR good practices for performance-based risk-sharing arrangements task force", *Value in Health*, Vol. 16 No. 5, pp. 703–719.

GKV-Spitzenverband (2019), *Kennzahlen der gesetzlichen Krankenversicherung*, Berlin.

Gonçalves, F. R., Santos, S., Silva, C. and Sousa, G. (2018), "Risk-sharing agreements, present and future", *Ecancermedicalscience*, Vol. 12 No. 823.

Jørgensen, J., Hanna, E. and Kefalas, P. (2020), "Outcomes-based reimbursement for gene therapies in practice: the experience of recently launched CAR-T cell therapies in major European countries", *Journal of market access & health policy*, Vol. 8 No. 1.

Levaggi, R. (2014), "Pricing schemes for new drugs: A welfare analysis", *Social Science & Medicine*, Vol. 102, pp. 69–73.

Lohmüller, J., Schröder, M. and Telschow, C. (2019), "Der GKV-Arzneimittelmarkt 2018: Trends und Marktsegmente", in Schwabe, U., Paffrath, D., Ludwig, W.-D. and Klauber, J. (Eds.), *Arzneiverordnungs-Report 2019: Aktuelle Daten, Kosten, Trends und Kommentare*, Springer Berlin, pp. 249–299.

Lorente, R., Antonanzas, F. and Rodriguez-Ibeas, R. (2019), "Implementation of risk-sharing contracts as perceived by Spanish hospital pharmacists", *Health Economics Review*, Vol. 9 No. 1, pp. 25–32.

Morgan, S., Grootendorst, P., Lexchin, J., Cunningham, C. and Greyson, D. (2011), "The cost of drug development: a systematic review", *Health policy*, Vol. 100 No. 1, pp. 4–17.

Neumann, P.J. (2013), "Where are we on 'risk-sharing' agreements?", *Value in Health*, Vol. 16 No. 5, pp. 701–702.

NICE (2002), *Technology Appraisal Guidance [TA32]: Beta interferon and glatiramer acetate for the treatment of multiple sclerosis*, London.

OECD (2010), *Value for Money in Health Spending, OECD health policy studies*, Paris.

Palace, J., Duddy, M., Bregenzer, T., Lawton, M., Zhu, F., Boggild, M., Piske, B., Robertson, N. P., Oger, J., Tremlett, H., Tilling, K., Ben-Shlomo, Y. and Dobson, C. (2015), "Effectiveness and cost-effectiveness of interferon beta and glatiramer acetate in the UK Multiple Sclerosis Risk Sharing Scheme at 6 years: a clinical cohort study with natural history comparator", *The Lancet Neurology*, Vol. 14 No. 5, pp. 497–505.

Palace, J., Duddy, M., Lawton, M., Bregenzer, T., Zhu, F., Boggild, M., Piske, B., Robertson, N. P., Oger, J., Tremlett, H., Tilling, K., Ben-Shlomo, Y., Lilford, R. and Dobson, C. (2019), "Assessing the long-term effectiveness of interferon-beta and glatiramer acetate in multiple sclerosis: Final 10-year results from the UK multiple sclerosis risk-sharing scheme", *Journal of neurology, neurosurgery, and psychiatry*, Vol. 90 No. 3, pp. 251–260.

Pearson, S. D., Thokala, P., Stevenson, M. and Rind, D. (2019), "The Effectiveness and Value of Treatments for Spinal Muscular Atrophy", *Journal of managed care & specialty pharmacy*, Vol. 25 No. 12, pp. 1300–1306.

Pfannstiel, M. A., Da-Cruz, P. and Schulte, V. (Eds.) (2019), *Internationalisierung im Gesund-heitswesen: Strategien, Lösungen, Praxisbeispiele*, Springer Gabler, Wiesbaden.

Renze-Westendorf, M. (2010), "Direktverträge als Instrument des Business-to-BusinessMarketings von forschenden Arzneimittelherstellern", in Loock, H. and Steppeler, H. (Eds.), *Marktorientierte Problemlösungen im Innovationsmarketing: Festschrift für Professor Dr. Michael P. Zerres*, Gabler Verlag, Wiesbaden, pp. 199–220.

Statistisches Bundesamt (Destatis) (2019), *Volkswirtschaftliche Gesamtrechnungen: Inlandsproduktberechnung - detaillierte Jahresergebnisse 2018, Fachserie 18, Reihe 1.4.*

Towse, A. and Garrison, L.P. (2010), "Can't get no satisfaction? Will pay for performance help? Toward an economic framework for understanding performance-based risk-sharing agreements for innovative medical products", *PharmacoEconomics*, Vol. 28 No. 2, pp. 93–102.

Vermeulen, K. M. and Krabbe, P. F. M. (2018), "Value judgment of health interventions from different perspectives: arguments and criteria", *Cost effectiveness and resource allocation*, Vol. 16 No. 16.

Including values and preferences
by patients in healthcare.
Methods and case studies

Integrating patients and social aspects into health technology assessment

Caroline Steigenberger / Petra Schnell-Inderst / Uwe Siebert

Abstract

This chapter describes how patients and the social perspective can be included in health technology assessments (HTA). Utilising an HTA is a common procedure for defining and describing the value of a health technology for health policy decision-making. The HTA reports are produced on medical interventions to map the value of a health technology for various stakeholders and serve as a basis for information. The evidence from the HTA report should enable health policy decision makers to decide whether or not a health technology should be approved and/or reimbursed.

The integration of the patient and social perspective into the evaluation process of health technologies is highly relevant in the health policy context. It provides an important contribution to understanding what the value of an intervention is for users. At the European level, the HTA Core Model®, which was developed by the European Network for HTA (EUnetHTA), offers a framework for orientation on how to elaborate the domain.

The aim of integrating patients and social aspects into the HTA report is to understand the needs, values and preferences of the users of a medical intervention better. The domain provides information on important facets of the value of a health technology for users, including moral values and information needs. Relevant outcomes are particularly the motivation in favour or against the intervention under investigation, access to, experience with and expectations of the intervention or to better understand possible unmet needs.

Nevertheless, the current state of the research is that although the inclusion of the patient perspective is considered an important issue by HTA agencies worldwide, there is a lack of implementation. The integration of patients is currently still rare and insufficiently systematic. Moreover, in most cases, there is no evaluation of the additional benefit of including patients or the patient perspective.

There are various ways to include the patient and social perspective in the HTA process. They can be included by either secondary data analysis or collecting primary data. The evidence can be qualitative or quantitative. A systematic elaboration of the patients and social aspects domain requires more resources in the production, but there are good reasons to elaborate the patient perspective and social aspects comprehensively. As an example of an HTA report with a focus on patients and social aspects, we describe the HTA commissioned by a German HTA agency on integrative mistletoe therapy for patients with breast cancer in addition to standard therapy.

In this project, it was already foreseeable before the start of the HTA project that there might be only a few randomised controlled trials on the effectiveness of mistletoe therapy in patients with breast cancer. If the evidence on effectiveness as a basis is unclear, it is difficult to make a recommendation. Nevertheless, mistletoe extracts are in demand. In order to understand better why this is the case, the patients and social aspects domain has also been systematically elaborated in this HTA report.

Although it is not possible to estimate what influence the results on patients and social aspects will have on health policy decisions, it is evident that the elaboration has provided valuable indications as to the value of mistletoe therapy for users.

Keywords: systematic review; patients and social aspects; health technology assessment (HTA); health policy decision-making; patient involvement

1 Valuation of health technologies

"What is the value of health interventions?" and "How to depict this value?" were the main questions that we discussed during the conference week. This chapter describes the empirical challenges that arise when patients and social aspects (SOC) are included in the evaluation of medical interventions in health technology assessments (HTAs). The topic is very relevant because it is important for decision makers to understand why patients, relatives and physicians want to have and use a medical intervention, sometimes even if the evidence base is insufficient to demonstrate clinical effectiveness or cost-effectiveness. Information on the experiences and expectations of health technology users in HTA reports can also be an important source of information for guideline authors to discuss these elusive aspects in guidelines.

1.1 What is health technology assessment?

After many years in which there was no internationally accepted definition of HTA, a joint task group, under the leadership of the International Network of Agencies for Health Technology Assessment (INAHTA) and Health Technology Assessment International (HTAi), has managed to create a definition of HTA for which there is a consensus on a global level. The new definition of HTA is as follows:

> HTA is a multidisciplinary process that uses explicit methods to determine the value of a health technology at different points in its lifecycle. The purpose is to inform decision-making in order to promote an equitable, efficient, and high-quality health system. (O'Rourke *et al.*, 2020, p. 2)

Four notes were added to clarify the meaning and scope of the definition in order to find a consensus among all institutions involved. The first note clarifies the broad scope of the term 'health technology':

> A health technology is an intervention developed to prevent, diagnose or treat medical conditions; promote health; provide rehabilitation; or organize healthcare delivery. The intervention can be a test, device, medicine, vaccine, procedure, program, or system. (O'Rourke *et al.*, 2020, p. 2)

The second note emphasises that the process has to be "formal, systematic, and transparent, and uses state-of-the-art methods to consider the best available evidence" (O'Rourke *et al.*, 2020, p. 2).

Regarding the definition of the value of medical interventions, the third note emphasises the many facets of the concept of value, which is composed of various dimensions:

> The dimensions of value for a health technology may be assessed by examining the intended and unintended consequences of using a health technology compared to existing alternatives. These dimensions often include clinical effectiveness, safety, costs and economic implications, ethical, social, cultural and legal issues, organizational and environmental aspects, as well as wider implications for the patient, relatives, caregivers, and the population. The overall value may vary depending on the perspective taken, the stakeholders involved, and the decision context. (O'Rourke *et al.*, 2020, p. 2)

The fourth note refers to the point in the life cycle of the evaluation. Health technologies are assessed via HTAs prior to or during their market access or within the process of re-evaluating an intervention which is already implemented as far as the stage of disinvestment of a health technology, in order to summarise the evidence currently available as a basis for decision-making by health policy decision makers (O'Rourke *et al.*, 2020).

1.2 Recommended domains for a health technology assessment

Before we describe how including SOC into an HTA report enables extra value for decision makers and patients in the end, it is important to understand how HTA reports are compiled. The systematic and transparent way of conducting an HTA is described in guidelines and handbooks. These documents usually also define the basic structure of the report. In addition, the methodology is mainly predefined and standardized.

Best practice recommendations of the European Collaboration in HTA (ECHTA) Working Group 4 (Busse *et al.*, 2002) suggest that an HTA should include a comprehensive background section describing the nature of the health problem with information on the burden of the disease, its epidemiology and who is the target population. Furthermore, the technology under assessment should be described and it should be stated at which point the technology stands in the product life cycle. In addition, alternative treatment options should be mentioned, including information on which treatment is currently the standard in practice.

There are five main domains that are relevant to consider (Busse *et al.*, 2002):

1. Safety
2. Efficacy/effectiveness
3. Psychological, social and ethical considerations
4. Organisational and professional implications
5. Economic issues

Recommendations from 2002 on which aspects to include in HTAs already contained psychological, social and ethical aspects as the main outcomes and an important part of HTA. Busse *et al.* (2002) stated that the correct way of approaching these aspects depends on the knowledge that is already available and may also comprise qualitative data or knowledge from other disciplines. The hierarchy of study designs describing the levels of evidence is not applicable to this domain (Busse *et al.*, 2002).

A more recent methodological framework is the HTA Core Model® (EUnetHTA, 2016a), which is a further development of the suggestions of the European Collaboration in HTA Working Group 4. The EUnetHTA HTA Core Model® (EUnetHTA, 2016a) was developed and refined during the EUnetHTA Project (2006–2008) and the two follow-up projects, EUnetHTA Joint Action (2010–2012), EUnetHTA Joint Action 2 (2012–2015), and during Joint Action 3 (2015–2021) (EUnetHTA, 2018). The project aim was to achieve a common understanding within Europe of what is a good methodology to generate an HTA report to facilitate collaborations across countries and enable efficient sharing of results.

Domains of the HTA Core Model® are (EUnetHTA, 2016a):

- Health problem and current use of technology (CUR)
- Description and technical characteristics of technology (TEC)
- Safety (SAF)
- Clinical effectiveness (EFF)
- Costs and economic evaluation (ECO)
- Ethical analysis (ETH)
- Organisational aspects (ORG)

- Patients and social aspects (SOC)
- Legal aspects (LEG)

It is noteworthy that the ethical analysis and the SOC part are divided into two different domains in the HTA Core Model®.

There are two types of HTA reports: rapid relative effectiveness assessments (REAs) and full HTA reports. An REA only includes the domains CUR, TEC, SAF and EFF, but full HTA reports comprise all nine domains when applicable to the health intervention assessed (EUnetHTA, 2020).

The HTA Core Model® (Version 3.0) (EUnetHTA, 2016a) is the current framework for European HTA collaboration. The production of joint REA reports should support a more efficient use of resources by avoiding duplication of work, because the same new health technologies are coming to the market in many European countries, which will usually be assessed by national HTA agencies. The joint REA reports are intended to be taken up in the national assessment.

European collaborations do not have the objective of making health policy decisions on a European level. The aim is for recommendations for reimbursement decisions to be made exclusively at a national level and that each country decides independently which services are to be integrated into the catalogue of healthcare services. The collaboration shall solely facilitate the exchange of evidence between HTA agencies that is applicable to different countries, such as evidence on effectiveness and safety. Domains, which can be different for different countries, will mainly be compiled for each country separately. It is suggested that a SOC domain is included on a national level.

1.3 The HTA Core Model® domain "Patients and Social aspects (SOC)"

The domain "Patients and Social aspects (SOC)" in the HTA Core Model® provides guidance on methodological issues arising when compiling the SOC domain (EUnetHTA, 2016b).

There are two main ways of integrating information on patients' aspects: (1) to summarise existing evidence in a secondary data analysis or (2) to gain primary data by conducting interviews or a survey. Both primary and secondary data analysis can be qualitative and/or quantitative. There are numerous different guidelines on how to conduct an HTA because each national HTA authority has its own handbook on how to conduct an HTA report properly.

In addition to different options of generating evidence on SOC, it is important to use a systematic and methodologically robust process for synthesizing and reporting the results. The SOC domain should be elaborated comparable to other domains to facilitate the integration of the domain into the HTA structure. However, neither a domain on social or ethical aspects nor qualitative evidence have been integrated into HTA reports in a standardized manner in the past, as described in section 03.1 (Merlin *et al.*, 2014).

There was a recommendation published by EUnetHTA in 2019 on how to integrate patient input in REAs (EUnetHTA, 2019), and this document is updated regularly. There are also initiatives that are constantly working to improve patient and public involvement and publishing guidance, such as the book by Facey *et al.* (2017) or the framework by Abelson *et al.* (2016).

How the integration of SOC is to be carried out according to the EUnetHTA Core Model® is described in more detail in sections 3.2, 3.3 and 3.4.

2. Why include patients and social aspects

Before we describe how SOC can be included in an HTA report and present an example of how we have integrated the domain into an HTA on the integrative mistletoe therapy in breast cancer patients, we explain why these aspects should be included.

2.1 The purpose of integrating patients and social aspects

Our HTA report is a practical example of how patient experiences influence the value of a technology.[1] In this chapter, we will not go into more detail about whether and why the patients and social perspective should be included, but we refer to the clear statement of the HTAi interest group for patient and citizen involvement, which sees great potential in the integration of the SOC domain. The interest group for patient and citizen involvement at HTAi states its position clearly on their website: "Vision: Patient and citizen perspectives improve HTA" (HTAi, 2020a).

In general, SOC should be integrated into HTA to understand the perspective of people affected by the health technology. The domain and the term "people affected" usually refers to patients (if necessary, represented by their parents or other relatives), individuals and caregivers (IQWIG, 2017b). Caregiv-

---

[1] A justification why patients' experiences should be taken into account when defining the value of a medical intervention is provided in another chapter of this book written by Ubels. He describes the value of additional information on patients' experiences on a theoretical level, in the context of the capability approach and how this could be integrated in practice. Including the patient perspective in decision-making is also the subject in Napiwodzka's ethical discussion of potentials and challenges for the Polish healthcare system in this volume.

ers come from the private environment of the patient, as family or friends, and are not healthcare professionals paid for the service (EUnetHTA, 2016b). The SOC domain provides information on what motivates patients to claim a treatment or intervention, respectively, what motivates individuals to use preventive interventions. Experiences regarding the impact of a health technology on everyday life and the perceived value of the quality and the benefit of the health technology can only be provided by those people affected (EUnetHTA, 2016b). Information on issues which promote or prevent a demand can also identify underlying unmet needs of the patients. Unmet needs can be diverse and may relate to information or social needs, uncertainty on the effectiveness and safety of a treatment, or limited access. The unmet needs are sometimes easy to meet, for example, if a patient wants to have the opportunity to discuss treatment options with a trusted doctor.

The SOC domain does not only include information on the motivation for using a certain health technology but also on how information is communicated to patients or where patients' needs, such as the need for information, are not met within the healthcare system (EUnetHTA, 2016b). Good counselling on a health technology, for example, improves the health literacy of the patient so that they can be a responsible decision maker regarding their own treatment process.

In addition to informing the patient about individual risks regarding the treatment, each therapy planning needs a benefit-risk assessment on an individual level before suggesting a therapy to the patient (Ernst and Klein, 2017). In case unmet needs arise that are related to patient information, communication, access to a treatment or other topics, the SOC domain would be the appropriate place to provide information on these aspects if available and suggest how to react adequately.

Since decisions on the implementation and refunding of health technologies are increasingly complex and have to be made under scarce resources, some countries (e.g. Australia) try to expand public engagement in order to create more transparency (Wortley et al., 2017).

A mapping review at EU level summarises the HTA processes of HTA agencies in Europe and describes similarities and differences in the approach leading to the creation of an HTA product (Chamova, 2017).

The German HTA agency Institute for Quality and Efficiency in Healthcare (IQWIG) involves patients in the dossier assessment (IQWIG, 2017a), in the suggestion (called "IQWIG ThemenCheck Medizin") and selection of topics for HTA, and offers the public the chance to react in written form on study plans and preliminary HTA reports (IQWIG, 2017b).

However, what is usually missing in HTA across different HTA agencies is the inclusion of the patients' perspective in the HTA report in the form of a literature review, as is done in other domains. To summarise the relevant evidence on SOC helps to represent the patients' perspective better.

Lehoux and Williams-Jones (2007) see an important responsibility of HTA agencies is to also constitute the diversity of social and ethical issues in addition to evidence on clinical and economic questions. Already addressing aspects as social justice and transparency in the HTA report helps decision makers to bring together public expectations, (moral) values, and evidence on effectiveness, safety and cost-effectiveness (Lehoux and Williams-Jones, 2007). A summary of existing evidence on the elusive topic of SOC makes it easier for decision makers to make sure they do not accidentally ignore important aspects.

2.2 Relevant outcomes for the patients and social aspects domain

The SOC domain in the HTA Core Model® contains eight assessment elements (see Table 1), which constitute the relevant outcomes for the domain. These assessment elements are assigned to three different thematic groups: patients' perspectives (which also include caregivers), social groups' aspects and communication aspects.

Topic	Assessment elements
Patients' perspectives	What are the experiences of living with the condition?
	What expectations and wishes do patients have regarding the technology and what do they expect to gain from it?
	How do patients perceive the technology under assessment?
	What is the burden on caregivers?
Social group's aspects	Are there groups of patients who currently don't have good access to available therapies?
	Are there factors that could prevent a group or person from gaining access to the technology?
Communication aspects	How are treatment choices explained to patients?
	What specific issues may need to be communicated to patients to improve adherence?

Table 1: Assessment elements for the patients and social aspects domain according to the EUnetHTA HTA Core Model® (EUnetHTA, 2016b, p. 348).

Some aspects may be irrelevant for the intervention under assessment, but each aspect should be checked for relevance. If it is not possible to answer all research questions, it is important to state which questions could not be answered based on the existing literature (EUnetHTA, 2016a).

3 How to include patients and social aspects

We will first consider the current situation since the extent to which SOC are included depends heavily on the commissioning HTA authority. Subsequently, we describe briefly how the creation of the SOC domain, as described in the HTA Core Model®, is carried out methodically as a systematic review.

3.1 Current state of including patients and social aspects

Despite the recommendations above, social aspects have often not been treated as a separate domain in the HTA report in the past. Two surveys – one paper-based survey in 2010 and one web-based follow-up survey in 2013 – were conducted within the 53, respectively, 56 member organisations of INAHTA to find out more about the core dimensions that are regularly used by HTA agencies (Merlin et al., 2014). A total of 45 (approximately 80 per cent) agencies participated in at least one survey. The participants were asked about their practice of including the nine different core domains – similar to those stated in the HTA Core Model®. The question should be answered regarding how likely it is that the institution addresses the respective area in the HTA product. An HTA product is, for example, a full HTA report, a rapid review or a mini-HTA. Regarding social aspects, 50 to 74 per cent of institutions answered that they generally include social aspects in full HTA reports (number of answers: 31). The inclusion of social aspects for HTA products with a smaller extent, such as a rapid review or a mini-HTA, is less than 25 per cent and may also be zero (Merlin et al., 2014).

Many HTA agencies in developed countries have standardized processes for the involvement of patients and the public. Patient engagement is described as important by several HTA societies, for example, HTAi, INAHTA or EUnetHTA (EUnetHTA, 2016b; HTAi, 2020b; Menon and Stafinski, 2011). Although patient and public participation (PPI) has increased in recent years, the effects of these initiatives were hardly evaluated by HTA agencies for a long time.

Nowadays, the involvement of patients is more established. A recent discussion paper published by Single et al. (2019) reports the opinion of experts on patient involvement from HTA agencies on the development and impact of patient involvement in HTA. Patient involvement had a positive impact in the institutions participating in terms of clarifying uncertainties and complementing clinical and economic evidence. The conclusion of the experts is that, so far, patient involvement has made a difference, especially in the recommendations on when and how the technology can be used (Single *et al.*, 2019).

A survey of the Patient and Citizen Involvement Group of HTAi with 15 responding HTA agencies (response rate of 27.8 per cent) tried to evaluate the potential usefulness of PPI initiatives. Fourteen respondents involved patients and ten involved the public in HTA. They recruited via the INAHTA and personal contacts. Approximately half of the institutions evaluated their PPI activities and used the insights to improve the activities and react on education and training needs (Weeks *et al.*, 2017). These results could indicate a gap in evaluating PPI initiatives in HTA agencies in general or that PPI initiatives are still neglected.

A specific example of the lack of including SOC in HTA, even when these aspects would be relevant for the assessment of the value of the intervention, is a knowledge synthesis by Potter *et al.* (2009) on how ethical, social and legal aspects (ELSI) are included in HTA for prenatal/preconceptional and newborn screening. The literature review and an associated workshop with different HTA agencies in which the findings were discussed showed that ELSI and public health ethics are highly relevant in the context of applying the screening intervention when they were taken into account. A second result was that ELSI have to be evaluated on a national level. The diversity between countries concerning cultural values, stakeholder communities and contextual factors need a flexible approach regarding how to address ELSI. Approaching ELSI should be adapted to each target population of the HTA (Potter *et al.*, 2009).

The authors of the publication criticise omitting elaborations on ELSI in HTA reports because it does not solve the problem that these aspects have to be considered when making the decision on reimbursing an intervention or permitting market access. It simply shifts the assessment of ELSI to a later stage in policy decision-making (Potter *et al.*, 2009). The more transparent the process is from excerpting study results on ELSI to the conclusions within an HTA report, the better health policy decision-making committees can justify their decision towards the public.

3.2 Gathering information

According to the SOC domain of the EUnetHTA HTA Core Model®, the methodology of how to elaborate the domain in a good practice depends on the existing knowledge on relevant outcomes. The relevant outcomes related to the health technology under assessment are stated in Table 1 (EUnetHTA, 2016b).

The process of defining the appropriate method starts with a literature search. If a current systematic review of patients' and social aspects has not yet been published, one has to be conducted. If the existing literature does not cover relevant aspects, an additional primary study can be conducted to solve the problem of missing information. Asking patient groups or patient organisations, for example, in focus groups is also an option (EUnetHTA, 2016b).

In practice, HTA agencies have to deal with limited budgets and the extent of patient involvement and how the domain shall be elaborated will be defined by the HTA agency that commissions the HTA.

3.3 Quality assessment of the studies included

The quality of the studies and reporting of the results within the publications for all studies included in the systematic reviews as part of an HTA has to be appraised to judge the strength of the evidence and enable transparency. One challenge is the huge amount of appraisal tools available for the critical appraisal of studies – as well as for qualitative and quantitative studies. A review conducted by Crowe and Sheppard in 2011 included 44 critical appraisal tools, of which five (11 per cent) included a comprehensive guideline on how to use the critical appraisal tool and how it was developed (Crowe and Sheppard, 2011). There was no test for reliability for 77 per cent of the appraisal tools and no information available about a validation of the tool for 25 per cent. Hence, the authors advise was to be careful when selecting and using an appraisal tool (Crowe and Sheppard, 2011). A mapping review on critical appraisal tools for qualitative studies shows a similar situation. Munthe-Kaas et al. (2018) conducted the mapping review with the aim of finding a critical appraisal tool that would be suggested for use in the GRADE-CERQual (Grading of Recommendations, Assessment, Development and Evaluations – Confidence in the Evidence from Reviews of Qualitative Research) assessment (Lewin et al., 2018). A total of 107 tools were identified, of which 40 have been published since 2010 (Munthe-Kaas et al., 2018). New tools do not usually refer to older tools or justify why a new tool was needed. The authors of the review conclude:

> the plethora of tools, old and new, indicates a lack of consensus regarding the best tool to use, and an absence of empirical evidence about the most important criteria for assessing the methodological limitations of qualitative research. (Munthe-Kaas et al., 2018, p. 1)

The Cochrane Qualitative and Implementation Methods Group (Noyes et al., 2018b) suggests using the checklists of the Critical Appraisal Skills Program (CASP) (CASP, 2018a, 2018b, 2018c, 2018d, 2018e).

There is no appraisal tool available in the CASP program for cross-sectional studies. Alternatively, two other checklists could be used: one tool is developed by Downes et al., the AXIS critical appraisal tool (2016), and the other is developed by the National Heart, Lung and Blood Institute (2020).

3.4 Analysing data on patients and social aspects

There are several methodological options to analyse the data, but we only present one option, which is commonly accepted in the literature (Higgins and Green, 2011; Noyes et al., 2018a). Both the qualitative and the quantitative research paradigm provide relevant information on SOC. Both types of data can be analysed separately and presented in the same chapter of the HTA report. If this option is chosen, the analysis of quantitative data is similar to evidence in other domains. Evidence is summarised, including relevant inferential and descriptive statistics, and presented in tables and narrative summaries.

Qualitative evidence is analysed by qualitative thematic synthesis, including a coding process, which is conducted by two independent researchers. "Coding" is the first step in a text analysis. The researcher reads the text line by line and summarises the meaning of a thematic unit in one word or phrase. This phrase is called "code". Both researchers must check the consistency of the interpretation of codes to make sure that the code depicts the meaning of what is said in the text. This check of consistency of the codes and the meaning of the text is repeated until both researchers agree. The second step is to deduce descriptive themes from the codes. This means that codes that are related to the same topic are merged into one descriptive theme. In a third step, the researchers must interpret the descriptive themes and make judgments on how the content of the descriptive themes can answer the research questions (Thomas and Harden, 2008).

4　Example: secondary data analysis on patients and social aspects in an HTA on mistletoe therapy in breast cancer patients

A focus on the SOC domain is still a special feature in HTA reports. One example for the elaboration of the SOC domain is the HTA report conducted recently on "Safety and efficacy of additional treatment with mistletoe extracts for patients with breast cancer compared to conventional cancer therapy alone", commissioned by the German Institute of Medical Documentation and Information (DIMDI) (Schnell-Inderst et al., 2020, under review). This report will presumably be public by the end of 2020. Previous assessments of mistletoe therapy in cancer patients hypothesized that there will be few studies available to assess safety, effectiveness and costs of a mistletoe therapy (Horneber et al., 2008; Kienle et al., 2009; Lange-Lindberg et al., 2006). However, mistletoe therapy has been used for many years. The section on SOC was elaborated in detail to understand why patients and doctors use additional mistletoe therapy and what they expect from it.

The HTA reports commissioned by DIMDI are often based on secondary data and systematic literature reviews or, in some cases, decision-analytic models. The contracting authority limits the sources of evidence to published literature, which has to be synthesized in a systematic review. We compiled the information regarding the SOC domain through a secondary data analysis of qualitative and quantitative studies.

4.1 Methods

A systematic literature research was performed to collect data for the secondary data analysis. A comprehensive search in medical databases (MEDLINE, EMBASE, Cochrane Library, the databases of the Centre of Reviews and Dissemination [DARE and HTA database], and CINAHL) was complemented by a search in databases from other disciplines, such as psychology, economics and social science, because medical databases probably do not contain all the relevant literature (Wessels *et al.*, 2016). The database search was supplemented by a comprehensive search on the internet. The "Grey Matters" tool, published by CADTH Information Services, has been used to identify grey literature (CADTH, 2015). Search terms included various different aspects related to the SOC domain and aspects related to complementary and alternative medicine (CAM) (Franzel *et al.*, 2013).

The inclusion criteria for the systematic review were:

- Population: patients with mammary carcinoma, their family caregivers, dependents, physicians and nurses
- Intervention: therapy with mistletoe extracts (subcutaneous, intravenous, in tumour tissue, in the gap between the lungs and pleura) additional to usual care (this has been extended to complementary and alternative medicine since there was scarce evidence on mistletoe therapy, but mistletoe therapy had to be reported separately)
- Outcomes: attitude and expectations towards, acceptance of, experiences and satisfaction with, knowledge about, access to and use of adjuvant mistletoe therapy; type, extent and evaluation of patient information and evaluation of the doctor-patient communication concerning adjuvant mistletoe therapy
- Study type: all study types were considered.

The check for eligibility of the papers was conducted by two independent authors. If the inclusion or exclusion of references was unclear, the authors solved discrepancies by discussion.

The study quality for the cross-sectional and qualitative studies has been assessed using the checklist for qualitative studies developed by the CASP Program (CASP, 2018c), as suggested by the Cochrane Qualitative and Implementation Methods Group Guidance (Noyes *et al.*, 2018b). Since there was no checklist available for cross-sectional studies when the systematic review was conducted, the checklist for cohort studies has been adapted by the research team of the HTA report (CASP, 2018b).

We analysed and reported the studies as described in section 3.4. The two qualitative studies were analysed in a thematic synthesis (Thomas and Harden, 2008) and quantitative evidence was summarised in tables. Both qualitative and quantitative results were narratively described, and the themes derived from the coding process were put together with the results from quantitative studies.

4.2 Brief preliminary results

Of the 302 publications screened in title and abstract, 84 were checked for eligibility in full text. A total of 13 publications were finally included in the analysis on SOC. Ten of the studies are from a patients' perspective, including two qualitative (Brandenberger *et al.*, 2012; Gschwendtner *et al.*, 2016) and eight quantitative (Drozdoff *et al.*, 2018; Fasching *et al.*, 2007; Fremd *et al.*, 2017; Huebner *et al.*, 2014; Moschen *et al.*, 2001; Schönekaes *et al.*; 2003, Tautz *et al.*; 2012, Templeton *et al.*, 2013) studies. Three studies focus on the physicians' perspective (Kalder *et al.*, 2001; Klein *et al.*, 2017; Muenstedt *et al.*, 2000).

All of the relevant outcomes that were stated in the inclusion criteria in section 4.1 have been addressed in the analysis within the HTA report. The main difference between our outcomes and those suggested in the SOC domain in the HTA Core Model® is a fourth main topic. In addition to patients', social groups' and communication aspects, the new topic is physicians' aspects. The analysis showed that physicians also had a broad range of experiences with, beliefs about and motivational causes in favour of or against mistletoe treatment.

In this book chapter, we can only address the results and challenges of the HTA report very briefly. For more information, please see the full HTA report by Schnell-Inderst *et al.* "Safety and efficacy of additional treatment with mistletoe extracts for patients with breast cancer compared to conventional cancer therapy alone", which is currently under review and going to be published by the DIMDI at the end of 2020. A summary in English will be available (Schnell-Inderst *et al.*, 2020, under review).

4.3 Discussion and challenges

The results of the SOC domain deliver valuable insights regarding the attitude towards and motivation in favour of or against supplementary mistletoe treatment. The results can enable decision makers to track medical decision-making on an individual level between physician and patient and enable responsible institutions to react to unmet information needs.

We faced some challenges related to the secondary data analysis on SOC related to the mistletoe therapy in breast cancer patients. Firstly, we had a problem due to the fact that mistletoe therapy was only addressed as one complementary treatment option of other complementary and alternative medicine in all quantitative studies from a patients' perspective. Therefore, we had to widen the scope of the intervention to integrative therapies in breast cancer patients. We included complementary and alternative medicine studies as long as mistletoe therapy was mentioned separately. This led to the next challenge, because the term "integrative medicine" has not yet been used in English publications but only "complementary medicine" or "complementary and alternative medicine". Unfortunately, up to now, the concept of complementary and alternative medicine is not clearly defined (Ernst and Klein, 2017) and comprises diverse supplementary treatments. Each study team defined for themselves which complementary and alternative medicine were to be included. This complicated the comparability and transferability of the results to the mistletoe therapy.

At this stage, it is not yet possible to estimate the impact of additional outcomes from the SOC domain. However, it has been confirmed that the evidence on efficacy, safety and cost-effectiveness available does not allow for a clear recommendation. The reasons for and against the use of integrative mistletoe therapy reflect the uncertainty among those treating and patients. At the same time, the results on SOC make it comprehensible why mistletoe extracts are, nevertheless, used and with what aim. Doctors might also find results from the SOC domain helpful in advising patients when they see that colleagues are equally unsure what to recommend and perhaps even that treatments are sometimes being performed with the sole purpose of motivating the patient. We are not saying that this cannot be a legitimate reason for using a form of therapy, but only that it is important to be aware of it.

In summary, in the authors' opinion, it made absolute sense to evaluate the SOC domain in detail in the HTA on integrative mistletoe therapy in breast cancer patients. The motivation of the patient or physician for the application of the mistletoe therapy is based on a broad spectrum of reasons, which represent the value for patients in various ways. If the evaluation had been based solely on the clinical and cost-effectiveness of mistletoe therapy, the value of mistletoe therapy for patients would probably not have been sufficiently understood.

References

Abelson, J., Wagner, F., DeJean, D., Boesveld, S., Gauvin, F. P., Bean, S., Axler, R., Petersen, S., Baidoobonso, S., Pron, G., Giacomini, M. and Lavis, J. (2016), "Public and patient involvement in health technology assessment: A framework for action", *International Journal of Technology Assessment in Health Care,* Vol. 32 No. 4, pp. 256–264.

Brandenberger, M., Simoes-Wüst, A. P., Rostock, M., Rist, L. and Saller, R. (2012), "Lebensqualität von Brustkrebspatientinnen während der Misteltherapie: Eine qualitative Studie", *Schweizerische Zeitschrift für GanzheitsMedizin,* Vol. 24 No. 2, pp. 95–100.

Busse, R., Orvain, J., Velasco, M., Perleth, M., Drummond, M., Gürtner, F., Jorgensen, T., Jovell, A., Malone, J., Ruther, A. and Wild, C. (2002), "Best practice in undertaking and reporting health technology assessments. Working group 4 report", *International Journal of Technology Assessment in Health Care,* Vol. 18 No. 2, pp. 361–422.

CADTH (2015), *Grey matters: A practical tool for searching health-related grey literature,* CADTH Information Services.

CASP (2018a), *CASP case control study checklist,* Oxford Centre for Triple Value Healthcare, Oxford. Available at: casp-uk.net/wp-content/uploads/2018/01/CASP-Case-Control-Study-Checklist-2018.pdf (accessed 2 December 2020).

CASP (2018b), *CASP cohort study checklist,* Oxford Centre for Triple Value Healthcare, Oxford. Available at: casp-uk.net/wp-content/uploads/2018/03/CASP-Cohort-Study-Checklist-2018_fillable_form.pdf (accessed 2 December 2020).

CASP (2018c), *CASP qualitative checklist,* Oxford Centre for Triple Value Healthcare, Oxford. Available at: casp-uk.net/wp-content/uploads/2018/01/CASP-Qualitative-Checklist-2018.pdf (accessed 2 December 2020).

CASP (2018d), *CASP Randomized Controlled Trial Checklist,* Oxford Centre for Triple Value Healthcare, Oxford. Available at: casp-uk.net/wp-content/uploads/2018/01/CASP-Randomised-Controlled-Trial-Checklist-2018.pdf (accessed 2 December 2020).

CASP (2018e), *CASP Systematic Review Checklist,* Oxford Centre for Triple Value Healthcare, Oxford. Available at: casp-uk.net/wp-content/uploads/2018/03/CASP-Systematic-Review-Checklist-2018_fillable-form.pdf (accessed 2 December 2020).

Chamova, J. (2017), *Mapping of HTA national organisations, programmes and processes in EU and Norway,* European Commission, Brussels.

Crowe, M. and Sheppard, L. (2011), "A review of critical appraisal tools show they lack rigor: Alternative tool structure is proposed", *Journal of Clinical Epidemiology,* Vol. 64 No. 1, pp. 79–89.

Downes, M. J., Brennan, M. L., Williams, H. C. and Dean, R. S. (2016), "Development of a critical appraisal tool to assess the quality of cross-sectional studies (AXIS)", *BMJ Open,* Vol. 6 No. 12.

Drozdoff, L., Klein, E., Kiechle, M. and Paepke, D. (2018), "Use of biologically-based complementary medicine in breast and gynecological cancer patients during systemic therapy", *BMC Complementary Medicine and Therapies,* Vol. 18 No. 1, p. 259.

Ernst, A. and Klein, S. (2017), "How to classify and evaluate complementary and alternative medicines in oncology [German]", *Deutsche Medizinische Wochenschrift,* Vol. 142 No. 12, pp. 873–881.

EUnetHTA (2016a), *HTA Core Model® Version 3.0 for the full assessment of diagnostic technologies, medical and surgical interventions, pharmaceuticals and screening technologies.* Available at: www.htacoremodel.info/BrowseModel.aspx (accessed 2 December 2020).

EUnetHTA (2016b), "Patients and social aspects (SOC)", in EUnetHTA Joint Action 2, Work Package 8 (Ed.), *HTA Core Model® Version 3.0*. Available at: www.htacoremodel.info/Browse Model.aspx (accessed 2 December 2020).

EUnetHTA (2018), *About EUnetHTA*. Available at: eunethta.eu/about-eunethta/ (accessed 2 December 2020).

EUnetHTA (2019), *Patient input in relative effectiveness assessments (Updated: 29 May 2019)*. Available at: eunethta.eu/wp-content/uploads/2019/06/Final_290519_Patient-Input-in-REAs.pdf (accessed 2 December 2020).

EUnetHTA (2020), *HTA Core Model®*. Available at: eunethta.eu/hta-core-model/ (accessed 2 December 2020).

Facey, K., Hansen, H. P. and Single, A. N. V. (2017), *Patient involvement in health technology assessment*, Springer Nature Singapore, Singapore.

Fasching, P., Thiel, F., Nicolaisen-Murmann, K., Rauh, C., Engel, J., Lux, M., Beckmann, M. and Bani, M. (2007), "Association of complementary methods with quality of life and life satisfaction in patients with gynecologic and breast malignancies", *Supportive Care in Cancer*, Vol. 15 No. 11, pp. 1277–1284.

Franzel, B., Schwiegershausen, M., Heusser, P. and Berger, B. (2013), "How to locate and appraise qualitative research in complementary and alternative medicine", *BMC Complementary Medicine and Therapies*, Vol. 13, p. 125.

Fremd, C., Hack, C. C., Schneeweiss, A., Rauch, G., Wallwiener, D., Brucker, S. Y., Taran, F. A., Hartkopf, A., Overkamp, F., Tesch, H., Fehm, T., Hadji, P., Janni, W., Luftner, D., Lux, M. P., Muller, V., Ettl, J., Belleville, E., Sohn, C., Schuetz, F., Beckmann, M. M., Fasching, P. A. and Wallwiener, M. (2017), "Use of complementary and integrative medicine among German breast cancer patients: predictors and implications for patient care within the PRAEGNANT study network", *Archives of Gynecology and Obstetrics*, Vol. 295 No. 5, pp. 1239–1245.

Gschwendtner, K. M., Holmberg, C. and Weis, J. (2016), "Beweggründe von Krebspatienten für und gegen die Inanspruchnahme der Misteltherapie", *Forschende Komplementarmedizin*, Vol. 23 No. 4, pp. 215–222.

Higgins, J. P. T. and Green, S. H. (2011), *Cochrane handbook for systematic reviews of interventions Version 5.1.0 [updated March 2011]*, The Cochrane Collaboration.

Horneber, M., Bueschel, G., Huber, R., Linde, K. and Rostock, M. (2008), *Mistletoe therapy in oncology*, The Cochrane Collaboration.

HTAi (2020a), *Patient and citizen involvement*. Available at: htai.org/interest-groups/pcig/ (accessed 2 December 2020).

HTAi (2020b), *Values and standards for patient involvement in HTA*. Available at: htai.org/interest-groups/pcig/values-and-standards/ (accessed 2 December 2020)

Huebner, J., Muenstedt, K., Prott, F. J., Stoll, C., Micke, O., Buentzel, J., Muecke, R., Senf, B. and Prevention, P. W. G. (2014), "Online survey of patients with breast cancer on complementary and alternative medicine", *Breast Care*, Vol. 9 No. 1, pp. 60–63.

IQWIG (2017a), *Involvement of people affected in the dossier assessment*. Available at: www.iqwig.de/download/Involvement-of-people-affected_dossier-assessment.pdf (accessed 2 December 2020).

IQWIG (2017b), *Beteiligung von Betroffenen bei der Erstellung von Berichten zur Nutzenbewertung*. Available at: www.iqwig.de/download/Betroffenenbeteiligung_Nutzenbewertungen.pdf (accessed 3 December 2020).

Kalder, M., von Georgi, R., Kullmer, U., Entezami, A., Hadji, P. and Munstedt, K. (2001), "Opinions of gynecologists on unconventional and complementary cancer therapy (UCT)", *Geburtshilfe Und Frauenheilkunde,* Vol. 61 No. 1, pp. 26–30.

Kienle, G. S., Glockmann, A., Schink, M. and Kiene, H. (2009), "Viscum album L. extracts in breast and gynaecological cancers: a systematic review of clinical and preclinical research", *Journal of Experimental & Clinical Cancer Research,* Vol. 28 No. 1, p. 79.

Klein, E., Beckmann, M. W., Bader, W., Brucker, C., Dobos, G., Fischer, D., Hanf, V., Hasenburg, A., Jud, S. M., Kalder, M., Kiechle, M., Kummel, S., Muller, A., Muller, M. T., Paepke, D., Rotmann, A. R., Schutz, F., Scharl, A., Voiss, P., Wallwiener, M., Witt, C. and Hack, C. C. (2017), "Gynecologic oncologists' attitudes and practices relating to integrative medicine: results of a nationwide AGO survey", *Archives of Gynecology and Obstetrics,* Vol. 296 No. 2, pp. 295–301.

Lange-Lindberg, A. M., Velasco-Garrido, M. and Busse, R. (2006), *Misteltherapie als begleitende Behandlung zur Reduktion der Toxizität der Chemotherapie maligner Erkrankungen [German],* HTA Report 44, German Institute of Medical Documentation and Information (DIMDI), Cologne.

Lehoux, P. and Williams-Jones, B. (2007), "Mapping the integration of social and ethical issues in health technology assessment", *International Journal of Technology Assessment in Health Care,* Vol. 23 No. 1, pp. 9–16.

Lewin, S., Booth, A., Glenton, C., Munthe-Kaas, H., Rashidian, A., Wainwright, M., Bohren, M. A., Tuncalp, O., Colvin, C. J., Garside, R., Carlsen, B., Langlois, E. V. and Noyes, J. (2018), "Applying GRADE-CERQual to qualitative evidence synthesis findings: introduction to the series", *Implementation Science,* Vol. 13 No. Suppl 1, p. 2.

Menon, D. and Stafinski, T. (2011), "Role of patient and public participation in health technology assessment and coverage decisions", *Expert Review of Pharmacoeconomics & Outcomes Research,* Vol. 11 No. 1, pp. 75–89.

Merlin, T., Tamblyn, D. and Ellery, B. (2014), "What's in a name? Developing definitions for common health technology assessment product types of the International Network of Agencies for Health Technology Assessment (INAHTA)", *International Journal of Technology Assessment in Health Care,* Vol. 30 No. 4, pp. 430–437.

Moschen, R., Kemmler, G., Schweigkofler, H., Holzner, B., Dunser, M., Richter, R., Fleischhacker, W. W. and Sperner-Unterweger, B. (2001), "Use of alternative/complementary therapy in breast cancer patients – a psychological perspective", *Supportive Care in Cancer,* Vol. 9 No. 4, pp. 267–274.

Muenstedt, K., Entezami, A. and Kullmer, U. (2000), "Oncologic mistletoe therapy – physicians use and estimated efficiency", *Deutsche Medizinische Wochenschrift,* Vol. 125 No. 41, pp. 1222–1226.

Munthe-Kaas, H., Bohren, M. A., Glenton, C., Lewin, S., Noyes, J., Tuncalp, O., Booth, A., Garside, R., Colvin, C. J., Wainwright, M., Rashidian, A., Flottorp, S. and Carlsen, B. (2018), "Applying GRADE-CERQual to qualitative evidence synthesis findings-paper 3: how to assess methodological limitations", *Implementation Science,* Vol. 13 No. Suppl 1, p. 9.

National Heart, Lung and Blood Institute, NIH (2020), *Study quality assessment tools: Quality assessment tool for observational cohort and cross-sectional studies,* U.S. Department of Health & Human Services, Bethesda, MD. Available at: www.nhlbi.nih.gov/health-topics/study-quality-assessment-tools (accessed 3 December 2020).

Noyes, J., Booth, A., Cargo, M., Flemming, K., Harden, A., Harris, J., Garside, R., Hannes, K., Pantoja, T. and Thomas, J. (2018a), "Chapter 21: Qualitative evidence", in Higgins, J., Thomas, J., Chandler, J., Cumpston, M., Li, T., Page, M. and Welch, V. (Ed.), *Cochrane hand-*

book for systematic reviews of interventions version 6.0 (updated July 2019), The Cochrane Collaboration, London.

Noyes, J., Booth, A., Flemming, K., Garside, R., Harden, A., Lewin, S., Pantoja, T., Hannes, K., Cargo, M. and Thomas, J. (2018b), "Cochrane Qualitative and Implementation Methods Group guidance series-paper 3: methods for assessing methodological limitations, data extraction and synthesis, and confidence in synthesized qualitative findings", *Journal of Clinical Epidemiology*, Vol. 97, pp. 49–58.

O'Rourke, B., Oortwijn, W., Schuller, T. and International Joint Task, G. (2020), "The new definition of health technology assessment: A milestone in international collaboration", *International Journal of Technology Assessment in Health Care*, Vol. 36 No. 3, pp. 187–190.

Potter, B. K., Avard, D., Entwistle, V., Kennedy, C., Chakraborty, P., McGuire, M. and Wilson, B. J. (2009), "Ethical, legal, and social issues in health technology assessment for prenatal/preconceptional and newborn screening: A workshop report", *Public Health Genomics*, Vol. 12 No. 1, pp. 4–10.

Schnell-Inderst, P., Steigenberger, C., Mertz, M., Otto, I., Flatscher-Thöni, M. and Siebert, U. (2020 [under review]), *Safety and efficacy of additional treatment with mistletoe extracts for patients with breast cancer compared to conventional cancer therapy alone [German]*, German Institute of Medical Documentation and Information (DIMDI), Cologne.

Schönekaes, K., Micke, O., Mucke, R., Buntzel, J., Glatzel, M., Bruns, F. and Kisters, K. (2003), "Anwendung komplementärer/alternativer Therapiemassnahmen bei Patientinnen mit Brustkrebs", *Forschende Komplementarmedizin und Klassische Naturheilkunde*, Vol. 10 No. 6, pp. 304–308.

Single, A. N. V., Facey, K. M., Livingstone, H. and Silva, A. S. (2019), "Stories of patient involvement impact in health technology assessments: A discussion paper", *International Journal of Technology Assessment in Health Care*, Vol. 35 No. 4, pp. 266–272.

Tautz, E., Momm, F., Hasenburg, A. and Guethlin, C. (2012), "Use of complementary and alternative medicine in breast cancer patients and their experiences: a cross-sectional study", *European Journal of Cancer*, Vol. 48 No. 17, pp. 3133–3139.

Templeton, A. J., Thürlimann, B., Baumann, M., Mark, M., Stoll, S., Schwizer, M., Dietrich, D. and Ruhstaller, T. (2013), "Cross-sectional study of self-reported physical activity, eating habits and use of complementary medicine in breast cancer survivors", *BMC Cancer*, Vol. 13 No. 1, pp. 1–8.

Thomas, J. and Harden, A. (2008), "Methods for the thematic synthesis of qualitative research in systematic reviews", *BMC Medical Research Methodology*, Vol. 8, p. 45.

Weeks, L., Polisena, J., Scott, A. M., Holtorf, A. P., Staniszewska, S. and Facey, K. (2017), "Evaluation of patient and public involvement initiatives in health technology assessment: A survey of international agencies", *International Journal of Technology Assessment in Health Care*, Vol. 33 No. 6, pp. 715–723.

Wessels, M., Hielkema, L. and van der Weijden, T. (2016), "How to identify existing literature on patients' knowledge, views, and values: the development of a validated search filter", *Journal of the Medical Library Association*, Vol. 104 No. 4, pp. 320–324.

Wortley, S., Tong, A. and Howard, K. (2017), "Community views and perspectives on public engagement in health technology assessment decision making", *Australian Health Review*, Vol. 41 No. 1, pp. 68–74.

The shared decision-making model and practical discourse to foster the appreciation of patients' value preferences in Polish healthcare

Discussing potentials and challenges

Karolina Napiwodzka

Abstract

The aim of the paper is to consider the potential and challenges regarding the implementation of the shared decision-making approach in the Polish health care system, also taking into account the moral and communicative-discursive advantages of such a change. The paper consists of several sections, in which the author: defines the objectives and method of the paper (Sections 1–2), presents the theoretical background of changes in health care (Section 3), and outlines the characteristics of Polish health care and the legal-institutional framework in Poland after the democratic turn in 1989 in terms of the ongoing communicative crisis in the relations between patients and health providers (Section 4). Next, the author distinguishes the ethical essentials of shared decision making, also presenting its affinities with J. Habermas' communication and discourse ethics, as an approach which can be applied in the clinical practice of medicine (Section 5), including the shared responsibility principle (Section 6). The next step was to name reasons for which health and medical values, SDM and practical discourse ethics can be linked together (Section 7). Then the author considers how the SDM model could be implemented through sampling cases from other countries (Section 8). Subsequently, she describes structural and normative potentials to adapt SDM and practical discourse ethics for Polish public health care (Section 9). A discussion follows.

Keywords: shared decision-making (SDM), communicative and discursive-ethical aspects of doctor-patient relationship, shared values and justified value and goal preferences in health care, Polish health care system, J. Habermas

1 Objectives

The main purpose of the paper is to consider the potential and challenges regarding the implementation of shared decision-making (SDM) in the Polish
healthcare system, taking into account the moral and communicative-
discursive advantages of such a change. The paper consists of several sections
which outline the SDM approach, revisit the core communicative-discursive
arguments that support it, weigh up the advantages and challenges of improving the SDM (also in terms of institutional framework and competencies), and
provide examples of its application to clinical practice.

While scholars highlight the need for patients' involvement in clinical
decision-making and report on related developments that have taken place in
countries across Central Europe, including Poland, after the democratic turn in
1989, some different developments can be observed: structural and compe-
tence-related barriers to communication and sharing clinical agreements and
decisions with patients, and discouraging patients from contributing to clinical
decision-making. Even though allowing patients to voice their concerns and
expectations is increasingly present in healthcare contexts, as is the practice of
healthcare providers listening to these perspectives, this alone is not equivalent to SDM, reciprocity and agreement. It is not the aim of this chapter to
evaluate these practices for economic value or effectiveness within
healthcare.[1] However, they certainly contribute to an area of shared health-
related values among patients and health professionals. How these values are
understood still remains a problematic question.[2]

2 Methods

The article reports on authors' investigations, supported by the topic-related
international literature, with a focus on the participation of patients in clinical
decision-making in the Polish context. The literature was used to 1) advocate
for the need of SDM and reciprocal agreement in clinical contexts and to 2)
describe and introduce the SDM approach as a socially inclusive method for
involving specific values, priorities and interests related to patients' health,
which already has the generally and publicly recognised status of one of the
core goods.

The data and selected literature on SDM are compared with Polish scholarship on the subject, within the specificity of Polish healthcare, and subsequently discussed. It is worth noting that the applicability of SDM varies with the

---

[1]   More on this perspective can be found, for instance, in Mitchell and Ubels in this volume.
[2]   For more on this subject, see Alex in this volume.

types of medical care (outpatient or inpatient care) and medical specialisations. Critical healthcare, for example, leaves little space for reciprocity, SDM and agreement, and refers more to healthcare providers' expertise and responsibilities. This paper revisits scholarship mainly referring to outpatient care, with the background of healthcare in general. The theoretical framework developed by the author focuses on communicative and discourse competences, actions and interactions as being supportive for SDM and agreement based on a shared *episteme*, the mutual understanding of the participants involved, and jointly discussed, weighed up, argued and justified outcomes, i.e. valid decisions and arrangements related to diagnosis, treatment and prophylaxis.

Within the framework of the communicative-discursive paradigm, the researcher intends to extract and analyse those moments of the communication situation where there is an exchange of arguments between at least two rational subjects who are able to speak to each other. One of the basic conditions for the occurrence of communicative and discourse interactions between the participants of clinical situations in which medical decisions, arrangements and agreements are made is that only such justifications that can be acceptable to all parties and reach an agreement are considered, while all the validity claims are maintained. The extensive international scholarship addressing the topic and reporting on developments and practices implemented elsewhere only confirms that the communicative and discursive 'state-of-the-art' in the Polish healthcare context is stunted when compared to other countries. However, the topic still remains a priority for international researchers and practitioners interested in the improvement of medical communication. Simultaneously, communication, discourse-based and SDM are becoming increasingly marginalised by new, technologically and digitally supported systems which tend to ease but also minimalize and marginalise the participation of human subjects. Unlike the recent technological approaches promoting electronic health (Gordon *et al.*, 2020; Sutton *et al.*, 2020),[3] this paper advocates improving the *human* and *interhuman* values and qualities of the practice of medicine.

3   Background

The primary goal of a healthcare system is to ensure that citizens have access to health services. From an ethical point of view, health is a special kind of good situated on the (social) border between the private and public, which makes it susceptible to institutional supervision, which is, in fact, necessary. Health as a social good and value is the subject of academic discussion, and

---

[3]   For recent investigations on interhuman medical communication, see Johnson (2019) and Hargraves *et al.* (2016).

each of the authors of this volume refers to it in some way.[4] The idea of fair and equal access to health services does not generally in itself raise moral objections. The problem arises when we try to clarify what 'health' and 'healthcare' mean, and what kind of health services people actually need and how to provide them.[5] Moreover, the specific organisation of the health-care system constitutes specific interpersonal relationships and social qualities between patients and medical professionals. In particular, chronic and long-term diseases have become a growing problem in Western societies. The distribution of goods in such diseases' related situations is often extremely challenging for decision makers.[6] However, the prevalence of chronic diseases also leaves some open room for models to involve patients' activism as decision makers. The area of inter-subjective interactions in medicine is particularly sensitive from the moral point of view and should be given careful consideration if a model of SDM, or something similar to it, is to be adopted.

The healthcare sphere is essentially that of interpersonal interactions and co-operation. This sphere differs from other social interactions and co-operation for several reasons. Firstly, it is the *vulnerability* of a living, human person into whose life healthcare providers make interventions through diagnosis and treatment. Such interventions are both actions and interactions: patients are not malleable material objects; their status and contributions are those of *subjects* who have their own personality, autonomy, rights, priorities and vital interests. Doctors' influence on patients might seem one-sided, as the former embody professional expertise and responsibilities, while the latter are laypeople, the passive recipients of healthcare provision and the charges of health providers. However, above and beyond such asymmetries, patients are very much involved in co-operating with these professional healers and carers. Co-operation is not just mechanical and economic (though contemporary healthcare systems improve marked-like relationships between healthcare contractors and purchasers). Interhuman co-operation implies that interaction is immediately managed by subjects in the process of communicating with another, to recognise the other, to understand each other and to make agreements and decisions at least with the patients' informed consent – if patients' active participation on medical decision-making is limited. The elements discussed above create a space for shared health-related values and preferences in medical contexts. According to the tradition and assumptions of the author of this chapter, these are values created and established through discourse and communication tools which will be described in more detail in the following paragraphs.

---

[4]   More on the health and disease definition in Stutzin Donoso in this volume.
[5]   More on justice and sustainable right to healthcare in Alex in this volume.
[6]   This is also addressed by Parsons in this volume.

The participants of such interaction (patients and their family members, healthcare providers, nursing personnel and further entitled agents) constantly have to manage a large and complex area of issues oscillating between life, health and well-being, one the one hand, and illness, pain, suffering, quality of life,[7] risk and mortality, on the other. Managing such a far-reaching and sensitive area which, additionally, touches patients' emotional and experiential sphere and their involvement in social reality (various *life-worlds* and *life forms*) seems to be unusually hard. Healthcare should, therefore, not only be reduced to the delivery of health services but should also embrace humanistic, social and communicative-discursive dimensions to allow the sharing of all kinds of related episteme and to open up an epistemic field or horizon within which healthcare professionals and patients meet together to communicate and develop decisions based on reciprocity and agreement. Within this intersubjective field, not only the existing scientific knowledge and medical expertise, evidence and *technai* are to be properly selected, agreed upon by subjects and applied. Novel knowledge, called "getting to know the patient" (Kępiński, 2002), which seems scarcely possible without the patient's contribution, is also produced here. Last but not least, clinical agreements and decisions rooted in this new knowledge should be shared, argued, justified and recognised by subjects who co-create their common field and intersubjective relationship within the field. The field is about reclassifying "a social logos into a *communicative dialogos*" (Siemek, 2000, p. 36), following M. J. Siemek, one of the leading advocates of applied intersubjectivity and practical discourse in Poland. "Effective doctor-patient communication is a central clinical function in building a therapeutic doctor-patient relationship, which is the heart and art of medicine. This is important in the delivery of high-quality health care" (Ha and Longnecker, 2010, p. 38).

A specific change can be identified as having occurred within the relationship patterns of healthcare providers and patients both on the international level and in Poland, reflecting changes that took place in bioethical reflection in the 20th century: a shift from the paternalistic model to informative or informed models and, finally, to deliberative or deliberation-supported modes.[8] Current models, taking into account practical needs, more or less fulfil the postulate of patient participation in the treatment process. However, the approach based on SDM seems to be closest to a full realisation of this postulate. Moreover, it has a number of advantages from the point of view of its therapeutic effectiveness and in terms of improving communicative-discursive qual-

---

[7]   More on this subject in Parsons in this volume.

[8]   The classical view of doctor-patients relationship models have been provided in Emanuel and Emanuel (2004). However, since that paper was published, a lot of sources have been found (it is not always about these "models" directly according to the classification mentioned above), for example, Gill *et al.* (2019), Inguaggiato *et al.* and Turabian (2019).

ity, which will be presented later in the paper. Considering primary care, several important issues may be highlighted. As Cheraghi-Sohi *et al.* noticed,

> Responding to the preferences of patients concerning, the delivery of health care is an important aspect of current health policy worldwide. This is especially relevant to primary care, which has traditionally been viewed as health care, which is oriented to the needs of patients rather than focused on technology. (Cheraghi-Sohi et al., 2006, p. 276)

As a part of primary care, medical professionals first contact patients (starting with the reception desk), which often sheds light on the rest of the therapy and treatment process (Légaré *et al.*, 2011; Meijers *et al.*, 2019).

4   Polish healthcare as an institution after the 1989 democratic turn

The Polish healthcare system is a part of the bigger sphere of public healthcare. According to the Polish Constitution, everyone has the right to have access to health care services, irrespective of their ability to purchase such services[9] (which may also be regarded in terms of A. Sen and M. Nussbaum's Capabilities Approach).[10] Health, as one of universally important social and individual values, goods and interests, is, thus, enshrined in the centre of social interest-sensitive legislation. On the one hand, health belongs to the key personal goods, however, on the other and, public supervision and protection is exercised over it. Models of healthcare are aimed precisely at such supervision and ensuring health protection as a value. However, the Polish healthcare system itself underwent radical reforms after 1989. A large number of social, economic, ethical, cultural and institutional factors have influenced its modernisation, including the democratic transformation in Poland, an unstable economic situation typical for post-communist countries, and the social and living conditions of the citizens during the transformation period.[11] Under the 1999 reform, the previous budget system (based on local health authorities, in Polish: *kasy chorych*) was replaced by the centralised insurance-budget system, which was based on the principle of social solidarity and the principle of uni-

---

[9]   "Everyone shall have the right to have his health protected. Equal access to health care services, financed from public funds, shall be ensured by public authorities to citizens, irrespective of their material situation. The conditions for, and scope of, the provision of services shall be established by statute" (The Constitution of the Republic of Poland, 1997).

[10]   For more on this perspective, see Mitchell and Ubels in this volume.

[11]   On the Polish healthcare system in the light of the transition and selected controversial issues connected to it, see Windak et al. (1998) and Nieszporska (2017).

versality. Established in 2004, the National Health Fund provides partial financing of health services from the taxpayers' public funds. The Polish healthcare system is currently based on general and mandatory social health insurance, but health services are increasingly simultaneously financed from private funds. Providing publicly financed health services (through the National Health Fund) is carried out through procedures. Service providers (medical facilities) could buy specific procedures that meet the health needs of the patients. However, it is assumed that there is no traditionally understood "healing process" within procedures (e.g. Piechota and Piechota, 2012; Śliwiński et al., 2013). The complexity and quality of the treatment/healing process depends not only on the type of procedures purchased and implemented by the facility. The issue is how these services are delivered: the emphasis is increasingly placed on efficiency and effectiveness and on efficient communication with patients.

It may be justified to refer to the changes which took place in Polish healthcare at the turn of the 20th and the 21st century as a communicative-discursive 'turn'. Not only have the organisational structures and methods of financing health services changed but also – perhaps above all – the relationships with stakeholders. There is a noticeable lack of encouragement to improve collaborative communication, reciprocity and shared agreement and decision-making in the Polish healthcare system, particularly regarding services financed from public funds. Scholars even report that there is a communication crisis or, at least, stagnation in the clinical relationships between healthcare providers and patients (Kuskowski, 2019; Schütte et al., 2018). Among the reasons for this, we could mention the arduous transition from the traditional (i.e. paternalistic) to modern (i.e. participatory) and patient-involving models of healthcare delivery (Emanuel and Emanuel, 2004; Sasz and Hollender, 1956), and deficits in the sphere of communicative-discursive models, practices and competences.[12] Communicational standards and decision-making practices have failed to keep up with modernisations and transformations triggered by the democratic turn after 1989. Although constantly undergoing reforms, healthcare provision in Poland shows that it lacks the capability and willingness to open itself to SDM and the emerging professional medical knowledge horizon with the social horizons represented by patients (DiMatteo, 1998; Greenfield et al., 1985; Lee and Garvin, 2003).

One of the most developed participatory models of the doctor-patient relationship is the SDM approach, which will be described briefly in the next section of the paper. The author recommends considering how such an approach could also work in the Polish healthcare area.

---

[12]   For more on the Polish healthcare difficulties, see Polak et al. (2019).

5 Ethical essentials of SDM with relations to discource ethics

Shared decision-making has been defined as "an approach where clinicians and patients share the best available evidence when faced with the task of making decisions, and where patients are supported to consider options, to achieve informed preferences" (Elwyn et al., 2012, p. 1361).

Firstly, taking into account autonomy as one of the most important ethical principles of modern medical ethics (Engelhart, 1986), priority is given to self-determination in this model. In the context of SDM, self-determination does not mean that individuals are abandoned.[13] Within this approach, the need to support autonomy is based on building good relationships, respecting both the individual competence and interdependence of others, and our intrinsic tendencies to protect and preserve our well-being. Elwyn and colleagues also use the term "relational autonomy" to articulate the statement, according to which "we are not entirely free, self-governing agents but that our decisions will always relate to interpersonal relationships and mutual dependencies" (Elwyn et al., 2012, p. 1361). Elwyn and colleagues' statement depicts *communicative intersubjectivity* as always being essential for, sensitive to and respecting other subjects' freedom and rights, which are fundamental for the practice of medicine as a social practice among autonomous and rational subjects – and crucial for patients' empowerment.

Secondly, SDM empowers patients' agency by providing high-quality information and supporting the decision-making process, for example, by means of deliberation,[14] There has been increasing emphasis on patient participation in the medical (clinical) decision-making process over the last few decades, (Frosch and Kaplan, 1999, p. 285).[15] Participatory models began to appear as an alternative to the paternalistic one in which the doctor makes all the treatment decisions. The patient's inclusion in the decision-making process began to be seen as necessary due to the emerging discursiveness of medicine (Rothman,

---

[13] "When offered a role in decisions, some patients feel surprised, unsettled by the offer of options and uncertainty about what might be best. If all responsibility for decision making is transferred to patients they may feel 'abandoned'. Some patients initially decline decisional responsibility role, and are wary about participating" (Elwyn *et al.*, 2012, p. 1363).

[14] Here the term 'deliberation' is used to "describe a process of considering information about the pros and cons of their options, to assess their implications, and to consider a range of possible futures, practical as well as emotional. [...] Deliberation begins as soon as awareness about options develops. The process is iterative and recursive, and the intensity increases after options have been described and understood" (Elwyn *et al.*, 2012, p. 1365).

[15] For recent applications of SDM, see: Bae (2017), Barrett *et al.* (2016), Knight (2019), Michalsen *et al.* (2019), Politi *et al.* (2013), Sommovilla *et al.* (2019) and Tamma *et al.* (2018).

1991). This tension between paternalistic and participatory models of healthcare delivery and the practice of medicine is particularly apparent in countries that have undergone political transformation (Antoun et al., 2011). A strong hierarchy in public services and asymmetry between 'laypeople' and 'professionals' was observed prior to the transition.

The principle of the patient's empowerment should not be confused (or be equated) with obtaining informed consent from a patient. As Frosch and Kaplan observed:

> While ethical guidelines mandate informed consent, especially when a recommendation involves a potentially harmful intervention, shared decision making goes several steps further. Beyond presenting the patient with facts about a procedure, shared decision making is a process by which doctor and patient consider available information about the medical problem in question, including treatment options and consequences, and then consider how these fit with the patient's preferences for health states and outcomes. After considering the options, a treatment decision is made based on mutual agreement. (Frosch and Kaplan, 1999, p. 285)

The communicative and discursive competencies of both the doctor and the patient are essential in the SDM process outlined above (Newton-Howes et al., 2019). There can be no question of formulating arguments as to a particular treatment path if the doctor is unable to formulate the judgments clearly and communicate them to the patient. Similarly, it is not possible to reach agreement on treatment if patients are unable to articulate their interests, preferences and needs.[16]

However, and this is the fourth point, this very basic, linguistic competence cannot be regarded as a communicative competence in Habermasian terms.[17] To Habermas, "language performance is an element of a monological capability" (1970) and, yet, not of a communicative ability or competence, respectively. To Habermas, communicative competence is originally and by definition *intersubjective and dialogical.*

The "basic qualifications of speech and symbolic interaction (role-behaviour) which we may call communicative competence" are required to develop communicative competence. "Thus communicative competence means the mastery of an ideal speech situation" (Habermas, 1970, p. 367) or – according to Habermas' concept of anticipating or approximating an ideal speech situation by real, socially embedded and world-situated participants – a skill to communicate interactively and consensually, i.e. oriented towards an agreement (*Verständigungsorientiertes kommunikatives Handeln*), within a communicative interaction with other subjects. Communication needs speech acts (Sprechakte), not just linguistic acts (Sprachakte). Furthermore, "I call interac-

---

[16] On patients who lack decision-making capacity, see Parsons in this volume.
[17] On Habermas' approach to medicine, see Habermas (1971, 1990) and Scambler (2001, 2015).

tions communicative when the participants coordinate their plans of action consensually, with the agreement reached at any point being evaluated in terms of the intersubjective recognition of validity claims" (Habermas, 1990, p. 58) of the proposed plans. Clarifying all 'yes' and 'no' statements, pros and cons, and the conditions of a rationally motivated agreement belongs to communicative interactions.

The uneven communicative skills of subjects (or their unequal rights to communicate) have dramatic consequences for communicative intersubjectivity: the "deformation of the intersubjectivity of mutual understanding which is built into the social structure" (Habermas, 1970, p. 372), including medical communication and the decision-making framework collaboratively made by patients and healthcare providers. Such a deformation implies further negative consequences for the reciprocal sharing, understanding and recognition of related interests, values and priorities and their validity (and validity claims).

It is worthwhile recalling Habermas' statement from the same book for the better inclusion of patients' cognitive perspectives and their interdependencies on their life-worlds and life forms as an integral content thematized within a communicative-intersubjective situation in clinical and medical contexts:

> The process of reaching an understanding between world and lifeworld. The lifeworld, then, offers both an intuitively preunderstood context for an action situation and resources for the interpretive process in which participants in communication engage as they strive to meet the need for agreement in the action situation. Yet these participants in communicative action must reach understanding about something in the world if they hope to carry out their action plans on a consensual basis, on the basis of some jointly defined action situation. (Habermas, 1970, p. 135)

Considering all four of the arguments in the check-list above, attention should also be given to the educational potential of communicative action and interaction, in Habermasian terms, for the implementation of the SDM approach in clinical contexts. According to Rusiecki and colleagues,

> Shared decision-making is a core competency in health policy and guidelines. Most U.S. internal medicine residencies lack an SDM education curriculum. A standardized patient (SP)-based curriculum teaching key concepts and skills of SDM was developed (Rusiecki et al., 2018, p. 1).[18]

---

[18] The Affordable Care Act has mandated that medical care include "shared decision-making programs between patients and physicians which incorporate the patient's preferences and values into the medical plan". The Accreditation Council for Graduate Medical Education echoes this sentiment, requiring residents to perform and incorporate SDM into their practice as an internal medicine milestone for effective patient communication. Despite these requirements, practitioners across all specialisations find the implementation of SDM into their daily practice difficult because of many barriers, including the lack of SDM training (Rusiecki et al., 2017).

On the one hand, this kind of communicative interpersonal practice is very suitable for recommendation in the practice of medicine as such, and the related skills should be implemented during the training of prospective medical professionals. On the other hand, patients should also be better trained in their communicative skills, so that they are enabled and empowered to participate in clinical communicative situations, such as SDM, whose outcomes require their agreement, usually practiced as simplified and under-considered forms of informed consent.

6   When A, then B? From shared decisions to shared responsibilities

Finally, both of the following are essential components of SDM: 1) communication and discourse ethics, with its key values and respect for patients' rights to voice their interests and priorities, to communicate in order to seek understanding, recognition and consensus, to participate in medical decisions and arrangements closely related to their health, etc., and 2) the ethical principle of responsibility ('shared responsibility'). Sharing responsibility unavoidably accompanies SDM, in the form of being actively engaged and participating in decision-making, achieving agreements and arrangements by means of communicative skills, and within intersubjective communication between healthcare providers and patients. All these activities can also be regarded as forms of self-determination and -governance assisted and supported by medical professionals' best expertise, evidence and scientific knowledge.

However, the principle of shared responsibility in medical decision-making contexts is also strictly connected to medical uncertainty, which is tied up with clinical practice. Responsibility belongs to the core values of healthcare delivery and medicine. However, one might ask if – and if so why – responsibility for choosing treatment and treatment outcomes should be shared between the doctor and the patient. The evaluation of available options for treatments and therapies must be based on the assessment of the patient's health condition (diagnosis). However, a patient also brings an important contribution to the discussion about the treatment options. Healthcare providers cannot access such information without conversation, i.e. knowing and properly understanding (and clarifying with a patient if necessary) the preferences regarding, for example, a patient's beliefs on well-being, health and risk, indications that someone leads an unhealthy or healthy lifestyle, their personal tolerances for pain and discomfort, their future plans and long-term health expectations, and prospects related to the therapeutic process and its dynamics, to prophylaxes, to plans (such as pregnancy), to professions, cultures and religions. (Frosch and Kaplan, 1999, p. 287). The communicative-discursive approach allows health professionals to learn more – and to become more mindful – about patients' individual value and goal preferences (see Section 9).

Responsibility in the healing process can manifest itself in various ways. In some cases, it may be limited to following the doctor's instructions (following a special diet, physical activity, taking prescribed medications regularly). In other cases, it concerns responsibility for the choice of treatment itself. The issue, particularly in the light of healthcare transitions, is the following: how to teach patients and sensitise them to this kind of shared responsibility? It is also one of the ethical issues in all relationship-centred models.[19]

To sum up this section, it should be stressed that the SDM approach is advantageous for several reasons. It requires the active participation and engagement of both the doctor and the patient, which is also relevant within the communicative-discursive paradigm. When patients actively participate in the treatment process, they are better prepared for following directions and have a better understanding of their health condition. From a medical point of view, it allows for better data collection and, thus, establishing optimal and effective treatment plans (it forces the doctor to consider all the treatment alternatives, therefore, the quality of decisions may be enhanced). Moreover, the SDM approach strengthens patients' autonomy through making them aware of the treatment decisions and the results and helps to develop shared responsibility for the treatment.

7   The appreciation of health and medical values in comparison to SDM in comparison to practical discourse

Since they deserve appreciation for their health-related values, patients involved in SDM (especially when linking this involvement with communication and discourse ethics) obtain a favourable opportunity to reorient healthcare providers' awareness and mindfulness – from the institutionalized and impersonal level of health and medical values 'in general', to the level of values (value preferences, respectively) which are to be actually determined for individual patients.

This opportunity would improve patients' health-related activism (Zoller, 2005) and, thus, their ability to express, co-determine and co-decide what matters or what is valid (in German *"was gilt"*) for them, since for Habermas, the decision-making process is value preference- and prior goal determination-laden. In communities with multiple values in which all subjects are potential patients, health-related preferences belong to the "strong preferences [...] that

---

[19]   On the relationship-centred approach, see Frankel (2004).

concern not merely contingent dispositions and inclinations but the self-understanding of a person". Unlike "weak or trivial preferences," strong preferences not only require "value decisions" but also "require justification" and "strong evaluations" and judgments, Habermas argues (1993, p. 4).[20]

As a consequence, the justification of patients' value and goal preferences necessarily implies patients' moral right to justification. Such a right is defended, for example, by R. Forst (2011). This right corresponds to the core premise of SDM, according to which SDM (similar to evidence-based medicine) aims at "the integration of best research evidence with clinical expertise and patient values" (Bae, 2017, s. 1.; Sackett *et al.*, 2000). Improving that right through SDM and practical discourse may advance the nature of clinical decision-making.

> In this regard, the shared decision-making model (SDM) is intended to replace the traditional style of asymmetrical one-way communication between physician and patient that has been handed down for centuries by medical tradition. (Kasper *et al.*, 2012, pp. 3–11)

The actualised and justified value preferences remain in resonance with the impersonal and universal values already framing healthcare – as one of the common social institutions. Additionally, involving both sides in SDM, i.e. healthcare providers and patients, combined with the communicative and discourse situation would provide more symmetry between the healthcare providers and patients' axiological perspectives regarding health improvement,[21] but also in the light of the unity of intersubjectively situated practical reason, pre-originally interested in sharing the values and normativities upon which subjects agreed or achieved an intersubjective *Verständigung* (understanding), respectively. The latter seems to be the very – and even only – source of values, regardless of these values to which a similar social agreement had already come into being previously (and still persists).[22] Finally, the appreciation of values by subjects involved in reciprocal, communicative and discourse relationships occurs through actual and factual confirmation vs. the questioning and disconfirmation acts performed by subjects with reference to their experience and practice ("*der Faktizität der kontextabhängigen und handlungsrelevanten Ja-/Nein-StellungnahmeI*") (Habermas, 1988, p. 182), especially

---

[20] In health and medical contexts, "the rational assessment of goals in the light of existing preferences" by several subjects – especially doctors and patients – is unavoidable. "Our will is already fixed as a matter of fact by our wishes and values; it is open to further determination only in respect of alternative possible choices of means or specifications of ends" (Habermas, 1993, p. 3).

[21] For social and axio-normative implications of perspective taking between "ego" and "alter" (*Perspektivenübernahme zwischen Ego und Alter*) and the idea of intersubjectivity, see Habermas (1988, pp. 178–185).

[22] On the controversy between value (what matters) vs. validity (what matters *and* is justified/righteous) in Habermas, see, for example, Harrington (2000, pp. 84–103).

from a patient. Maintaining a link to a patient's lived and actual values and their vital interests is essential for applying SDM and practical discourse in order to make the treatment as appropriate and beneficial for them as possible, i.e. to balance health values between the needs and demands arising from someone's actual health condition, on the one hand, and the health, well-being and further common values upheld by the healthcare system as a common social institution serving all, on the other hand. The intersubjective aspect of value appreciation within medical and clinical contexts gives saliency to what Habermas names "solidarity" (*solidarisches Zusammenwirken*) among the subjects making up a society and being concretely (*nicht in abstracto*) oriented towards relieving the plights of fellow creatures and implementing their intended priorities.[23]

In the following section I will consider in which clinical circumstances it may be possible and adequate to implement SDM (and related elements of practical discourse ethics) within clinical practice.

8   How can SDM and practical discourse models be implemented? Sampling cases

Generally, given the possibility of implementing relationship-centred models (in the broad sense) for clinical practice, the following question emerges: do we have any framework for this? According to Frosch and Kaplan,

> several conditions must be met for shared decision making to occur. First, the atmosphere must be conducive to active patient participation. The attending physician must make patients feel that their contributions are valued. Patients in turn need to be frank about their preferences and goals for treatment. The physician then helps the patient determine how these goals and preferences fit with the available treatment options and a shared decision is reached. (Frosch and Kaplan, 1999, p. 285)

These conditions should also include the communicative-discursive competences which are essential for functioning in public life area in general.

The most important issue for many practitioners is how the idea of SDM can work in daily clinical practice. Elwyn *et al.* (2012) formulated a three-step, simplified model for clinical practice which consists of several parts: choice, option and decision talk. As the authors observe,

> Choice talk refers to the step of making sure that patients know that reasonable op-

---

[23]   "[...] *kooperativer Anstrengung, die Leiden versehrbarer Kreaturen zu mildern, abzuschaffen, oder zu verhindern*" (co-operative effort to alleviate, abolish, or prevent the suffering of vulnerable creatures) (Habermas, 1988, p. 186).

tions are available. Option talk refers to providing more detailed information about options and decision talk refers to supporting the work of considering preferences and deciding what is best. The model outlines a step-wise process, although it is important to recognise that the model is not prescriptive – clinical interactions are by necessity fluid. Decision support tools provide crucial inputs into this process. (Elwyn et al., 2012, p. 1363)

There is still no guidance in Polish healthcare on how to implement SDM elements in medicine. However, it could be interesting to consider in what clinical circumstances the doctor can really makes decisions with the patient.

As a meaningful example, one may consider hypertension as one of the conditions that is typical and widely present in the literature.[24] This is a condition in which close co-operation between the doctor and the patient is necessary. The therapy will have no effect without patient involvement: elimination of drugs, changes in lifestyle and taking medication. However, this is not all that can be said about the patient's participation in the treatment process in this case. Some interventions may have long-term benefits while reducing the quality of life in the short term. Recalling Frosch's example, a patient with mild hypertension may experience no symptoms now, but taking anti-hypertensive pharmacotherapy may cause symptoms in the form of side effects. However, this therapy may lead to overall better life expectancy. Reducing the long-term morbidity associated with the consequences of hypertension is the aim of such therapy. On the other hand, reduced blood pressure does not necessarily imply certain long-term health benefits. As a result, the gain from taking anti-hypertensive medication is delayed and probabilistic (Frosch and Kaplan, 1999, p. 285). In a case like this, it is necessary for the doctor to be able to talk to the patient and present all the possible side effects and the expected effects of the therapy exhaustively. However, it is also important for the patient to bring information into the discussion about their preferences, life plans that may affect therapy and any significant claims about the treatment.

More straightforward and readable examples from oncology can be found. In the already classic article on the subject, Charles and colleagues outline three scenarios in which a patient with newly diagnosed early breast cancer shares the best treatment options with her physician (Charles et al., 1997, p. 691). As a part of this model example, we can see how the doctor guides the patient through the decision-making process, taking her concerns, preferences and wishes into account. In this case, effective decision-making is recommended because of the need to choose the treatment path quickly. It will be completely different, for example, in the case of chronic diseases, such as diabetes.

---

[24] Research findings in UK, US: Johnson et al. (2018). See also Langford et al. (2019). Another interesting example may be diabetes care, see Marker et al. (2018).

9 SDM meets Polish healtcare system: open questions

Considering the implementation of SDM elements in such systems as Polish healthcare, two basic research questions can be posed: firstly, are patients sufficiently encouraged and empowered and competent (in terms of Habermas' communicative competence and related competences described in this article) to actively and effectively participate in and contribute to clinical and medical decisions concerning their health?

Secondly, and this may be even more relevant, do doctors want patients to make decisions? As far as the former question is concerned, one can once again notice the tension between the paternalistic and participatory models in medicine. Patients sometimes simply do not want to participate in the treatment process for various reasons. They intuitively feel, for example, that the doctor should be the only decision maker because of his/her expertise and professional skills or, alternatively, they are afraid of taking the responsibility that would emerge with participation in the treatment process. According to Elwyn's general findings,

> some healthcare professionals express doubts, saying that patients don't want to be involved in decisions, lack the capacity or ability, might make 'bad' decisions, or worry that SDM is just not practical, given constraints such as time pressure. Others claim they are 'already doing it', though data from patient experience surveys indicates that this is not generally the case. It is therefore clear that the first step for those advocating the uptake of SDM is to ensure that clinicians and others support the underlying rationale. (Elwyn *et al.*, 2012, p. 1362)

Similarly, in Polish society, the tension between citizens' participatory needs and their 'paternalistic' habits or expectations can be observed, especially in elderly people who still remain mentally rooted in the past reality (pre-democratic, social, political and institutional) which was much less favourable for an individual's participation in decision-making. Polish people are becoming more active when communicating with doctors due to open access sources on the Internet, the availability of medical knowledge and their health awareness. However, both reliable research on the issue and in-depth reflection in interdisciplinary teams are still needed. When it comes to the second question – do doctors want patients to make decisions? – the attitudes of doctors can vary significantly (Hall *et al.*, 2018).

Several difficulties may be identified within the public part of the healthcare system including the lack of time for consultation, staff shortages, financial limits for tests, long waiting time for highly specialised care and difficulties in accessing specialised tests. In turn, another group of issues involves the limited discursive competences of stakeholders (limited discursive competences in the public sphere in general), communication disturbances and interaction misunderstandings. It is also worth noting that there is general dissatisfaction regarding the public healthcare system. The majority of patients are dissatisfied with the quality of services. The number of patients' grassroots initiatives (Borek and Chwiałkowska, 2014) has also been increasing in recent years.

The question remains open regarding what kinds of clinical decision-making (considering the difficulties mentioned above) are most amenable to being transformed into decision-making that involves patients. Is the Polish healthcare system itself suitably designed to enable SDM? One of the ideas for improving the quality of services was the legal act on primary care in 2017.[25] According to this idea, the primary care physician (family doctor or internist) was to play the role of a patient's 'guide' in the world of the complex dependencies of health services (this is particularly useful when a doctor meets a patient for the first time). The continuity and comprehensiveness of activities for the patient was emphasised within this idea. The diagnostic and therapeutic procedure offered the opportunity to get to know the patient better and share some decisions.

Apart from a group of factors directly related to the provision of medical procedures (diagnostic and therapeutic), one can consider the challenges that Polish healthcare has to face in order to be able to implement more patient- or relationship-centred solutions, such as SDM. One of the important, broader issues is how to share responsibility among doctors and patients. This happens when doctors motivate patients, to make them empowered and mobilized, not passive and dependent; when patients have the opportunity to verbalise and define their emotions, the patients' concerns are taken into account in the diagnosis and establishing the treatment plan, and when doctors accept that there is a need for equal communicative competence between themselves and their patients, because the expert knowledge of doctors is not enough to make the decision that is best for their patients.

Finally, one should consider, especially in the light of intensive changes in healthcare, how to educate doctors and patients in the area of communicative and moral-discursive competences. Medical simulation centres are a relatively new method of educating physicians in terms of communication with patients. Thanks to training involving role-playing in specific clinical situations, medical students and professionals can acquire the practical skills necessary to provide information to patients and their families. However, it should be noted that providing information is only one aspect of communication with patients. Communicative-discursive competences require the equal participation of the doctor and the patient in the treatment process, which is also important in the SDM approach. This aspect should be given more attention in future research.

---

[25] In Polish: Ustawa o podstawowej opiece zdrowotnej z dn. 27 października 2017 r., Dz.U. 2017, poz. 2217.

10 Conclusions and further research perspectives

Shared decision-making is an advantageous and valuable approach, widely described in international scientific scholarship and successfully implemented in clinical practice in several countries. Its implementation requires meeting basic institutional and organisational conditions, and the competences of the participants of clinical interaction. As a result, this approach would contribute to strengthening patients' empowerment and self-determination. Moreover, from the ethical point of view, it could help to create a common area of shared, health-related values in medicine. Many elements of practical discourse are implemented within SDM. The participants of the interaction can learn from each other how to understand the other person's views and how to agree upon value and goal preferences. Both the expertise and axiology of health professionals differ (or may differ, as shown above) from the expertise, and value and goal preferences embodied by patients (Leanza *et al.*, 2013). Including the latter in clinical decision-making supported by SDM and practical discourse ethics would improve patients' right to justification and their participatory contributorship, which was the subject of Section 7.

When considering SDM elements in daily clinical practice in Poland, several challenges must be considered: (1) have we already achieved sufficient institutional and infrastructural conditions for relationship-centred approaches? (2) How can the communicative-discursive competences of patients and healthcare providers be improved to increase the participatory and dialogical style of communication in clinical contexts, as communication resulting in shared decisions, justifications and agreements being made. (3) In what clinical circumstances would patients' more active contribution to the treatment, diagnosis and prophylaxes-related decisions be most appropriate and which systems and procedures would support it, as healthcare has many sectors and organisational and management levels.

It is difficult to answer these questions and to estimate the chances for the adoption of SDM in the Polish healthcare system. Episodic pathbreaking activities undertaken by patients can be observed (Drozd-Garbacewicz, 2015; Molęda, 2011; Napiwodzka, 2020 in process; Nowak *et al.*, 2020, in process). In the light of the communicative-discursive and participatory-deliberative turn in healthcare delivery systems observed in numerous countries (though not in all), the SDM approach has been underrepresented in Polish medical-ethical scholarship until now. I hope that this article makes a preliminary contribution to its consideration in Poland and discussing challenges related to this subject in the international context.

References

Antoun, J., Phillips, F., and Johnson, T. (2011), "Post-Soviet transition: Improving health services delivery and management", *Mount Sinai Journal of Medicine*, Vol. 78, pp. 436–448.

Barrett B., Ricco J., Wallace M., Kiefer D., and Rakel D. (2016), "Communicating statin evidence to support shared decision-making", *BMC Family Practice*, Vol. 17 No. 41.

Bae, J.-M. (2017), "Shared decision making: Relevant concepts and facilitating strategies", *Epidemiology and Health*, Vol. 39, e201748.

Beauchamp, T. L., and Childress, J. F. (2001), *Principles of biomedical ethics*, Oxford University Press, New York.

Borek, E., and Chwiałkowska, A. (2014), "Partycypacja pacjentów w procesie podejmowania decyzji w ochronie zdrowia w Polsce [Patients participation and shared decision-making in the polish healthcare system]", *Journal of Health Sciences*, Vol. 4 No. 1, pp. 289–296.

Charles, C., Gafni, A., and Whelan, T. (1997), "Shared decision-making in the medical encounter: What does it mean? (or it takes at least two to tango)", *Social Science & Medicine*, Vol. 44, pp. 681–692.

Cheraghi-Sohi, S., Bower, P., Mead, N., McDonald, R., Whalley, D., and Roland, M. (2006), "What are the key attributes of primary care for patients? Building a conceptual 'map' of patient preferences", *Health Expectations*, Vol. 9, pp. 276–284.

DiMatteo, M. R. (1998), "The role of the physician in the emerging healthcare environment", *Western Journal of Medicine*, Vol. 168 No. 5, pp. 328–333.

Drozd-Garbacewicz, M. (2015), "Współczesna rola pacjenta hospitalizowanego w interakcji z lekarzem – między konfliktem a równowagą", Doctoral Dissertation, Gdansk University.

Emanuel, J. E., and Emanuel, L. L. (2004), "Vier Modelle der Arzt-Patient Beziehung," in: Wiesing, U. (Ed.), *Ethik in der Medizin*, Reclam, Stuttgart.

Engelhart, T. H., (1986), *The Foundations of Bioethics*, Oxford, New York.

Elwyn, G., Frosch, D. L., and Kobrin, S. (2016), "Implementing shared decision-making: Consider all the consequences", *Implementation Science*, Vol. 11, p. 114.

Elwyn, G., Frosch, D., Thomson, R., Joseph-Williams, N., Lloyd, A., Kinnersley, P., Cording, E., Tomson, D., Dodd, C., Rollnick, S., Edwards, A., and Barry, M. (2012), "Shared decision making: A model for clinical practice", *Journal of General Internal Medicine*, Vol. 27 No. 10, pp. 1361–1367.

Forst, R. (2011), *The right to justification: Elements of a constructivist theory of justice,* trans. by J. Flynn. Columbia University Press, New York.

Frankel, R. M. (2004), "Relationship-centered care and the patient-physician relationship", *Journal of General Internal Medicine*, Vol. 19 No. 11, pp. 1163–1165.

Frosch, D. L., and Kaplan, R. M. (1999), "Shared decision making in clinical medicine: Past research and future directions", *American Journal of Preventive Medicine*, Vol. 17 No. 4, pp. 285–294.

General Medical Council U.K. (2008), Consent: Patients and doctors making decisions together (guidance for doctors). Available at: https://www.gmc-uk.org/-/media/documents/gmc-guidance-for-doctors---consent---english_pdf-48903482.pdf (accessed 3 December 2020).

Giersdorf, N., Loh, A., Bieber, C., Caspari, C., Deinzer, A., Doering, T., Eich, W., Hamann, J., Heesen, C., Kasper, J., Leppert, K., Müller, K., Neumann, T., Neuner, B., Rohlfing, H., Scheibler, F., van Oorschot, B., Spies, C., Vodermaier, A., Weiss-Gerlach, E., Zysno, P., and

Härter, M. (2004), "Entwicklung eines Fragebogens zur Partizipativen Entscheidungsfindung", *Bundesgesundheit - Gesundheitsforschung - Gesundheitsschutz*, Vol. 47, pp. 969–976.

Gill, S. D., Fuscaldo, G., and Page, R. S. (2019), "Patient-centred care through a broader lens: Supporting patient autonomy alongside moral deliberation", *Emergency Medicine Australasia*, Vol. 31 No. 4, pp. 680–682.

Gordon, W. J., Landman, A., Zhang, H., and Bates, D W. (2020), "Beyond validation: Getting health apps into clinical practice", *Digital Medicine*, Vol. 3 No. 14.

Greenfield, S., Kaplan, S., and Ware, J. E. Jr. (1985), "Expanding patient involvement in care. Effects on patient outcomes", *Annals of Internal Medicine*, Vol. 102 No. 4., pp. 520–528.

Ha, J. F., and Longnecker, N. (2010), "Doctor-patient communication: A review", *Ochsner Journal*, Vol. 10 No. 1, pp. 38–43.

Hall, K. H., Michael, J., Jaye, C., and Young, J. (2018), "General practitioners' ethical decision-making: Does being a patient themselves make a difference?", *Clinical Ethics*, Vol. 13 No. 4, pp. 199–208.

Habermas, J. (1970), "Towards a theory of communicative competence", Inquiry, Vol. 13, pp. 361–362.

Habermas, J. (1971), "Vorbereitende Bemerkungen zu einer Theorie der kommunikativen Kompetenz", in: Habermas, J. and Luhmann, N. (Ed.), *Theorie der Gesellschaft oder Sozialtechnologie,* Suhrkamp, Frankfurt am Main.

Habermas, J. (1988), *Nachmetaphysisches Denken*, Suhrkamp, Frankfurt am Main.

Habermas, J. (1990), *Moral consciousness and communicative action,* trans. Ch. Lenhardt, Weber Nicholsen, S., introduction by McCarthy, T., Polity Press, Cambridge.

Habermas, J. (1993), *Justification and application*, trans. Cronin, C., The MIT Press, Cambridge, Mass./London, England.

Hargraves, I., LeBlanc, A., Shah, N. D., and Montori, C. M. (2016), "Shared decision making: The need for patient-clinician conversation, not just information", *Health Affairs*, Vol. 35 No. 4, pp. 627–629. doi: 10.1377/hlthaff.2015.1354.

Harrington, A. (2000), "Value-spheres or validity-spheres? Weber, Habermas and modernity," *Max Weber Studies,* Vol. 1 No. 1, pp. 84–103.

Inguaggiato, G., Metselaar, S., Molewijk, B., and Widdershoven, G. (2019), "How moral case deliberation supports good clinical decision making", *AMA Journal of Ethics,* Vol. 21 No. 10, pp. 913–919.

Johnson, R. A., Huntley, A., Hughes, R., Cramer, H., Turner, K. M., Perkins, B., and Feder, G. (2018), "Interventions to support shared decision making for hypertension: A systematic review of controlled studies", *Health Expectations*, Vol. 21 No. 6, pp. 1191–1207.

Johnson, T. (2019), "The importance of physician-patient relationships communication and trust in health care", Duke Center for Personalized Healthcare. Retrieved from https://dukepersonalizedhealth.org/2019/03/the-importance-of-physician-patient-relation ships-communication-and-trust-in-health-care/ (accessed 2 December 2020).

Kasper, J., Légaré, F., Scheibler, F., and Geiger, F. (2012), "Turning signals into meaning – 'shared decision making' meets communication theory", *Health Expectations*, Vol. 15, pp. 3–11.

Kępiński, A. (2002), „*Poznanie chorego* [*Getting to know the patient*]", Wydawnictwo Literackie, Kraków.

Knight, K. (2019), "Who is the patient? Tensions between advance care planning and shared decision-making", *Journal of Evaluation in Clinical Practice*, Vol. 25 No. 6, pp. 1217–1225.

Kuskowski P. (Ed.), (2019), *Doświadczenia pacjenta w Polsce: raport badawczy Siemens Healthineers [Patient's experience in Poland: Research report Siemens Healthineers]*, Warszawa.

Leanza, Y., Boive, I., and Rosenberg, E. (2013), "The patient's lifeworld: Building meaningful clinical encounters between patients, physicians and interpreters", *Community Medicine,* Vol. 10 No. 1, pp. 13–25.

Lee, R. G., and Garvin, T. (2003), "Moving from information transfer to information exchange in health and health care", *Social Science and Medicine,* Vol. 56 No. 3, pp. 449–464.

Légaré, F., Stacey, D., Pouliot, S., Gauvin, F.-P., Desroches, S., Kryworuchko, J., Dunn, S., Elwyn, G., Frosch, D., Gagnon, M.-P., Harrison, M. B., Pluye, P., and Graham, I. D. (2011), "Interprofessionalism and shared decision-making in primary care: A stepwise approach towards a new model", *Journal of Interprofessional Care,* Vol. 25 No. 1, pp. 18–25.

Marker, A. M., Noser, A. E., Clements M. A., and Patton S. R. (2018), "Shared responsibility for type 1 diabetes care is associated with glycemic variability and risk of glycemic excursions in youth", *Journal of Pediatric Psychology,* Vol. 43 No. 1, pp. 61–71.

Meijers, M. C., Noordman, J., Spreeuwenberg, P., Hartman, T. C., and van Dulmen, S. (2019), "Shared decision-making in general practice: An observational study comparing 2007 with 2015", *Family Practice,* Vol. 36 No. 3, pp. 357–364.

Michalsen, A., Long, A. C., DeKeyser, G. F, White, D. B., Jensen, H. I., Metaxa, V., Hartog, C. S., Latour, J. M., Truog, R. D., Kesecioglu, J., Mahn, A. R., and Curtis, J. R. (2019), "Interprofessional shared decision-making in the ICU: A systematic review and recommendations from an pxpert Panel", *Critical Care Medicine,* Vol. 47 No. 9, pp.1258–1266.

Molęda, S., "Pacjent w wieku 16 lat współdecyduje o swoim zdrowiu [A 16-year old patient collaboratively decides on his own health]", *Puls Medycyny,* May 11, 2011. Retrieved from https://pulsmedycyny.pl/pacjent-w-wieku-16-lat-wspoldecyduje-o-swoim-zdrowiu-888858 (accessed 2 December 2020).

Napiwodzka, K. (2020, in process), *"Communicative action and practical discourse to empower patients in healthcare-related decision making",* Folia Philosophica Universitatis Lodziensis.

Newton-Howes, G., Pickering, N., and Young, G. (2019), "Authentic decision-making capacity in hard medical cases", *Clinical Ethics,* Vol. 14 No. 4, pp. 1–5.

Nieszporska, S. (2017), "Priorities in the Polish health care system", *European Journal of Health Economics,* Vol. 18, pp. 1–5.

Nowak, E., Mazur, P., and Napiwodzka, K. (2020, in process), "Prawo pacjenta do informacji w ujęciu komunikacyjno-dyskursywnym [Patient's right to information from a communicative-discursive perspective]".

Piechota, A., and Piechota, M. (2012), "Adult intensive therapy services contracted by the National Health Fund in 2012", *Anesthesiology Intensive Therapy,* Vol. 44 No. 3, pp. 123–129.

Polak, P., Świątkiewicz-Mośny M., and Wagner, A. (2019), "Much ado about nothing? The responsiveness of the healthcare system in Poland through patients' eyes", *Health Policy,* Vol. 123 No. 12, pp. 1259–1266.

Politi, M. C., Wolin, K., and Légaré, F. (2013), "Implementing clinical practice guidelines about health promotion and disease prevention through shared decision making", *Journal of General Internal Medicine,* Vol. 28 No. 6, pp. 838–844.

Rothman, D. J. (1991), *Strangers at the bedside: history of how law and bioethics transformed medical decision making,* Basic Books, New York.

Rusiecki, J., Schell, J., Rothenberger, S., Merriam, S., McNeil, M., and Spagnoletti, C. (2018), "An innovative shared decision-making curriculum for internal medicine residents: Findings from the University of Pittsburgh Medical Center", *Academic Medicine,* Vol. 93 No. 6, pp. 937–942.

Sackett, D. L., Straus, S. E., Richardson, W. S., Rosenberg, W., and Haynes, R. B. (2000), *Evidence-based medicine: How to practice and teach EBM,* 2nd ed. Churchill Livingstone, Edinburgh.

Sasz, T. S., and Hollender, M. H. (1956), "The basic models of the doctor-patient relationship", *Archives of Internal Medicine*, Vol. 97, pp. 585–592.

Scambler, G. (2001), "System, lifeworld and doctor–patient interaction. Issues of trust in a changing world", in: Scambler, G. (Ed.), *Habermas, critical theory and health*, Routledge, London/New York.

Scambler, G. (2015), "Jürgen Habermas: Health and healing across the lifeworld-system divide", in Collyer, F. (Ed.), *The Palgrave Handbook of Social Theory in Health, Illness and Medicine*, Palgrave Macmillan, London, pp. 355–369.

Schütte, S., Acevedo, P. N. M., and Flahault, A. (2018), "Health systems around the world – a comparison of existing health system rankings", *Journal of Global Health*, Vol. 8 No. 1, p. 010407.

Siemek, M. J. (2000), "Two models of dialogue", *Dialogue & Universalism*, Vol. 11, p. 3755.

Śliwiński, Z., Frączek, E., and Starczyńska, M. (2013), "Role of the physiotherapist in the orthopaedic trauma department in the context of National Health Fund funding of medical procedures", *Ortopedia, Traumatologia, Rehabilitacja*, Vol. 15 No. 6, pp. 629–639.

Sommovilla, J., Kopecky, K. E., and Campbell, T. (2019), "Discussing prognosis and shared decision-making", *Surgical Clinics of North America*, Vol. 99 No. 5, pp. 849–858.

Sutton, R. T., Pincock, D., Baumgart, D. C., Sadowski, D. C., Fedorak, R. N., and Kroeker, K. I. (2020), "An overview of clinical decision support systems: Benefits, risks, and strategies for success", *Digital Medicine*, Vol. 3 No. 17.

Tamma, P. D., Miller, M. A., and Cosgrove, S. E. (2018), "Rethinking how antibiotics are prescribed", *Journal of the American Medical Association*, Vol. 321 No. 2, pp. 139–140.

The Constitution of the Republic of Poland of 2nd April, 1997, Dziennik Ustaw, No. 78, item 483, article 68. Retrieved from https://www.sejm.gov.pl/prawo/konst/angielski/kon1.htm (accessed 2 December 2020).

Turabian, J. L. (2019), "Doctor-patient relationships: A puzzle of fragmented knowledge", *Journal of Family Medicine and Primary Care*, Vol. 3 No. 128, pp. 1–7.

Windak, A., Tomasik, T., and Kryj-Radziszewska, E. (1998), "The Polish experience of quality improvement in primary care", *The Joint Commission Journal on Quality Improvement*, Vol. 24 No. 5, pp. 232–239.

Death or dialysis: the value of burdensome life-extending treatments for the cognitively impaired

Jordan A. Parsons

Abstract

All medical treatments carry with them some level of burden for the patient, though this is usually outweighed by the benefits. Some long-term, life-extending treatments, however, are highly burdensome and the benefits are not always clearly greater. When a patient lacks decision-making capacity, there is a risk of undue harm if the decision is made on their behalf to initiate that treatment. In this chapter, I question the prioritisation of life-extension over quality of life in such circumstances, arguing that the latter ought sometimes to be prioritised. I suggest that in appealing to the principle of equal treatment of the cognitively impaired (which is endorsed in the majority of countries and is often the very purpose of legislation which governs treatment decisions for this population) we ought to accept that the very fact some patients with decision-making capacity choose to forego a medical intervention entails that sometimes cognitively impaired patients in similar situations ought also to forego that medical intervention. In doing so, maintenance dialysis is employed as a case study.

Kidney failure is a reality for millions of individuals globally. Due to the shortage of organs for transplantation, patients with or approaching kidney failure are usually started on maintenance dialysis. This is often considered the default, with the alternative of conservative kidney management – which, incidentally, some studies have suggested may provide a similar survival benefit in some patients – thought of as giving up. Dialysis is a hugely burdensome treatment, often proving both physically and mentally exhausting and thereby negatively impacting on quality of life. Depending on treatment modality it may also require thrice weekly visits to an outpatient unit for the procedure to be performed. With the increasing age of the dialysis population, for patients to have several comorbidities is common and may compromise quality of life further. Given the significance of these burdens, it is not uncommon for patients – particularly those who are older and with several comorbidities – to forego dialysis in favour of conservative kidney management.

Many of the burdens associated with dialysis may be exacerbated in cognitively impaired patients; they may not understand why they are being put through the treatment, and dialysis clinics may not be suitable environments depending on the nature of the patient's impairment. Not only are the burdens high for cognitively impaired patients, but these patients may be subjected to them for an extended period of time. The organ shortage, as well as many older cognitively impaired patients not being suitable candidates for transplantation, mean that dialysis is not always a bridge therapy. Rather, it is something that will be a part of the rest of these patients' lives. This raises the question of dialysis withdrawal, which I frame in terms of the equivalence thesis and the possible omission bias of clinicians.

I conclude that given some patients choose themselves to forego dialysis, patients who lack decision-making capacity ought sometimes also to forego dialysis in favour of conservative kidney management. This discussion is applicable to other highly burdensome treatments for cognitively impaired patients, and indeed is also useful in considering decisions concerning dialysis more broadly. Nonetheless, I also call for further research in this area to better explore the issues raised.

Keywords: Dialysis, Conservative kidney management, Kidney failure, Cognitive impairment, Dementia, Ethics

1   Introduction

All medical interventions entail some level of burden to the patient, whether as trivial as the inconvenience of adhering to a course of antibiotics or as significant as the lengthy recovery time following major surgery. These burdens are usually justified on the basis of being outweighed by the benefits of the intervention which, in general, means the curing of the patient's ailment or at least the relief of symptoms. Some interventions, however, are not so clearly justified on this basis; sometimes the burdens seem equal to – perhaps even greater than – the benefits. Providing treatments with apparently greater burden than benefit is not ethically problematic if the patient has provided properly informed consent following discussion of available options.[1] However, where a patient lacks decision-making capacity[2] there is a risk of them being significantly burdened without sufficient benefit-related justification.

---

[1]   In the interests of patient autonomy, patients have a right to make what may seem to an observer to be bad decisions. There is disagreement as to the limits of this right, but that is beyond the scope of this chapter.

[2]   Use of the term 'decision-making capacity' in this chapter refers to a patient's lack of decision-making capacity specifically in relation to the decision as to whether to initiate

In this chapter, my focus is long-term, life-extending medical interventions which are recognised as highly burdensome. As a case study, I will discuss the value of maintenance dialysis for adult patients with or approaching kidney failure[3] who lack decision-making capacity. This is a pertinent example given the extent of the burden dialysis entails; it is an intervention which continues on a regular basis for decades in many cases, and, for most, until death.

The starting point of this discussion is that a decision as to the initiation of dialysis for a cognitively impaired patient must be made, and must be made in that patient's best interests.[4] Of course, it is possible that such a patient will have previously formally expressed views which a doctor is unsure as to whether to respect. There may be concerns over when the views were expressed or what information they were based on (Conneen et al., 1998; Scott et al., 2018). This represents a voluminous discussion in its own right and will not, therefore, be discussed here. Rather, it will be assumed that no such views have been previously expressed by the patient.[5]

It is not my intention in this chapter to provide an answer as to whether a cognitively impaired patient should be started on dialysis. Indeed, I do not believe it is appropriate to seek such a blanket solution since decisions of this nature will be highly individualised to each patient.[6] Instead, I will demonstrate that cognitively impaired patients should *sometimes* forego dialysis through a discussion of quality of life concerns and the role of dialysis as a bridge therapy. This will appeal to the principle of equal access to healthcare for the cognitively impaired. First, though, I will provide some background to kidney failure and its treatment.

For patients with or approaching kidney failure, there are few options: transplantation, dialysis, or conservative kidney management (CKM). The pre-

---

maintenance dialysis. Decision-making capacity is decision specific so a patient who lacks the capacity to consent to dialysis may still be able to make other decisions about their care and/or non-health matters.

[3] Chronic kidney disease is considered to become kidney failure when it reaches Stage 5, which is the point at which the patient's estimated glomerular filtration rate drops below 15ml/min/1.73m2 (National Institute for Health and Care Excellence, 2015).

[4] The term 'best interests' has a specific legal meaning in some countries – notably in England and Wales where it is an important element of the Mental Capacity Act 2005. The use of the term in this chapter, whilst inevitably bearing similarities to this legal meaning, is more general and ethical and should not be interpreted strictly in line with the Mental Capacity Act 2005 usage or that of any other legislation.

[5] It is, of course, preferable for there to be previously expressed preferences of the patient to guide the decision-making process. As such, patients who can ought to be encouraged to make views and preferences known as early as possible (meaning upon being diagnosed with chronic kidney disease) in case they later lose cognitive function. That way supported decision making is more likely to be feasible which is preferable in terms of respect for autonomy to any form of substitute/proxy decision maker.

[6] For further discussion of the individualised nature of medical decisions in relation to wider obligations to society, see the chapter in this volume by Alex.

ferred option is a kidney transplant, though the global shortage of organs for transplantation means that this is often not an option. Even if a patient is likely to receive a transplant, waiting lists are usually several years. It is therefore common for patients to dialyze as a bridge therapy when the long-term plan for their care is a transplant, essentially leaving two choices for most patients with or approaching kidney failure: dialysis or CKM.

There are several dialysis modalities. The more traditional haemodialysis requires a patient to sit for a period of four hours, three times a week, connected to a dialysis machine through an arteriovenous fistula or other type of vascular access. This can be done at home, though it more often requires attendance at an outpatient unit. Peritoneal dialysis, on the other hand, is usually done at home. Dialysate is left in the abdominal cavity for a period of time before it is drained, and this is usually done several times daily or can be done by machine overnight. As it does not require the patient to frequent a dialysis centre, peritoneal dialysis is generally considered to allow greater independence and may, therefore, be best suited to patients who are more active.

The alternative, non-dialytic pathway is CKM. The intention of CKM is to ease symptoms and, at least to some extent, preserve kidney function. Many elements of CKM, such as dietary changes and medications, are also part of the care of a patient who is receiving dialysis; indeed, both options are much the same aside from the dialysis itself. CKM is not intended as a long-term option, but rather as end-of-life care. For patients who choose to forego dialysis, CKM will generally provide several months of life (O'Connor and Kumar, 2012), though this can be considerably less depending on the patient's situation. It is, therefore, an option mostly chosen by patients who are elderly and/or have severe comorbidities.

Among chronic kidney disease (CKD) patients, cognitive impairment is more prevalent than in those with normal kidney function. This is especially true of those who have progressed as far as Stage 3 of five (Torres *et al.*, 2017). Studies have also shown that cognitive function declines more rapidly in CKD patients (Findlay *et al.*, 2019), which is likely a result of the high burden of vascular disease. As such, more than 30% of patients established on dialysis have severe cognitive impairment (Ying *et al.*, 2014).

What makes this particular discussion necessary is the concern that some nephrologists favour dialysis to too great an extent (Jha *et al.*, 2017). Of course, the reverse will be true for some, as found by the Conservative Kidney Management Assessment of Practice Patterns Study (Roderick *et al.*, 2015). This is equally problematic, though it is more often reported that dialysis is overused than underused. The combination of the availability of dialysis and the technological imperative[7] is causing the overuse of dialysis, and arguably a loss of

---

[7]   There are several conceptions of the technological imperative. Its use in this chapter relates to Fuchs' definition as "giving the best care that is technically possible" (Fuchs,

focus on patients' quality of life in favour of length of life (Ying *et al.*, 2014). Favouring one care option is not itself problematic, but it has been found to negatively affect the decision-making process. Kaufman and colleagues have reported that some patients feel dialysis was not a choice they made, but it just "happened" (Kaufman *et al.*, 2006, p. S180). These patients had decision-making capacity and still found themselves on dialysis almost as a matter of procedure, so for patients who are unable to consent there is a risk that dialysis will be initiated when it is not clearly appropriate.

To avoid confusion, it is worth noting that I am concerned only with *maintenance* dialysis[8] for *adult* patients. Thus, any use of 'dialysis' should be read as 'maintenance dialysis', and 'patient(s)' as 'adult patient(s)'. Maintenance dialysis for children raises further value questions, as does acute dialysis for any patient. Whilst this discussion will certainly apply to some aspects of these other decisions, they differ in ways too significant to discuss here.

Further, I am concerned only with *permanently* cognitively impaired patients.[9] In the context of maintenance dialysis, as opposed to emergency dialysis, there is rarely an urgency to decisions; the condition of a patient is unlikely to decline with such a pace that an immediate decision is necessary. Therefore, if a patient has fluctuating decision making capacity, it would generally be appropriate to delay the decision – within reason and clinical feasibility – to allow the patient to make the decision. If it is necessary that the decision to initiate dialysis be made in the best interests of a patient with fluctuating decision-making capacity, that patient may regain decision-making capacity and at that point choose to withdraw dialysis. This is important as decision-making capacity is decision specific (MacPhail *et al.*, 2015), so the inability of a patient to consent to the initiation of dialysis does not necessarily preclude that same patient from consenting to the later withdrawal of dialysis.

2 Quality of life

Quality of life is a common thread to discussions of the value of medical interventions. In health economics, it has long been a guiding principle in assessing the cost-effectiveness of treatments (MacKillop and Sheard, 2018). The approp-

---

1968, p. 192). This is taken to mean extending life if possible – an attitude of "I can, so I should". This is, of course, partially attributable to societal pressures.

[8]   As opposed to emergency dialysis for the treatment of acute kidney disease. Whilst some of this discussion will be relevant to decisions concerning emergency dialysis, it is not my focus.

[9]   Arguably, certainty as to the permanence of a patient's cognitive impairment is not always possible as patients can and do unexpectedly regain cognition. Nonetheless, for the purposes of this discussion a patient is deemed permanently cognitively impaired when there is no clinical expectation that they will regain cognition.

riateness of quality-adjusted life years (QALYs) as a measure is contested yet it continues to guide healthcare commissioning decisions.[10] The role of quality of life in *ethical* discussions, however, is less contentious. The burdens of an intervention have just as important a role in decision making as its benefits. It is, however, not a simple calculation as with QALYs, as it is a more nuanced consideration.

Dialysis is a burdensome intervention. Not only does it take its toll physically on the body of the patient, but it can be mentally exhausting too. For some patients (particularly those that are cognitively impaired) further physical toll may come from the need to be physically and/or chemically restrained to provide dialysis; it is not uncommon for patients on dialysis to be physically resistant (O'Dowd *et al.*, 1998).[11] Further, there is a social burden given the time commitment and the potential strain a patient's dialysis schedule might have on relationships with loved ones. In some cases, patients receiving haemodialysis have suffered posttraumatic stress disorder as a result of their care (Tagay *et al.*, 2007). However, it is important to note variation in the impact dialysis has on patients. For some, the burden is perceived as minimal, with the lives of many patients on dialysis being only marginally inconvenienced. It seems trite to say that all patients have different experiences of the same treatment, but this is very much the case with dialysis.

The nature and extent of the burden of dialysis can vary significantly with treatment modality. Haemodialysis is generally considered more burdensome than peritoneal dialysis due to the more frequently necessary visits to outpatient units (Li *et al.*, 2010). As earlier noted, peritoneal dialysis is more common among younger patients with kidney failure who lead active lifestyles. For patients on peritoneal dialysis, the burden is likely to lie primarily in the side-effects, such as fatigue and peritonitis (National Health Service, 2018). For those on haemodialysis,[12] frequent visits to an outpatient unit may prove more burdensome given dialysis-related fatigue.

Patients with kidney failure are usually on a high number of medications, in part because of comorbidities. A 2009 study found the high pill burden of patients with kidney failure to be associated with a lower quality of life (Chiu *et al.*, 2009). Indeed, the median pill burden was 19, exceeding 25 in some participants. This may increase when being treated for infections at the site of the patient's arteriovenous fistula or catheter, which are common (Nassar and Ayus, 2001).

Dialysis, then, is burdensome, at least to some extent, for all patients. For

---

[10] See the chapters by Ubels and Mitchell in this volume for further discussion of the capability approach as an alternative.
[11] Dialysis patients may be noncompliant in a variety of ways, including physical resistance, missed sessions, and a failure to adhere to necessary dietary restrictions.
[12] Assuming they attend an outpatient unit for haemodialysis, which is most common.

those with significant comorbidities, however, the burden is often intensified. With the average age of patients on dialysis rising, comorbidities – notably hypertension – are increasingly common. A 2015 study, for example, found that 40% of (mostly older) participants with Stage 3 CKD had three or more comorbidities (Fraser *et al.*, 2015). Whilst haemodialysis can prolong life in the over-75s, it has been found that high comorbidity compromises this survival benefit. This is especially true of those with heart disease (Murtagh *et al.*, 2007). Further, patients with dementia prior to starting haemodialysis do particularly poorly, with an average time to death of 1.09 years, and 2-year survival rate of 24% compared to 66% in patients on dialysis without dementia according to a 2006 study (Rakowski *et al.*, 2006).

Some comorbidities may cause mobility issues which are especially problematic for patients undergoing haemodialysis at an outpatient unit. One such patient explained in an interview; "I've got an ulcerated leg, and my legs give way, and I am so frightened that I am going to fall" (Noble *et al.*, 2009, p. 86). Given the frequency of visits required for haemodialysis, mobility issues will inevitably exacerbate the burden of dialysis. This is a particular issue for patients in their eighties and nineties, for whom the combination of frequent visits and mobility issues may worsen the fatigue experienced.

Concerns have also been raised as to the suitability of the environment in which haemodialysis takes place, as it may be "dementia unfriendly" due to being an unfamiliar environment that may be noisy and busy, as well as a possible lack of continuity of staff (MacPhail *et al.*, 2015, p. 492). This is in addition to the need to tolerate invasive equipment whilst sitting still for long periods of time. Whilst this study concerned patients with dementia, the same concerns hold true for patients who are cognitively impaired in other ways.

Compared to dialysis, CKM generally has a lesser burden and resultant decrease in quality of life. This is because many burdens faced by patients on dialysis are a result of the dialysis itself. However, CKM does still carry some burdens. As earlier noted, CKM entails much the same care as that received by a patient on dialysis, the difference being the absence of dialysis. Therefore, pill burden remains an issue for conservatively managed patients. Whilst similar efforts are made in CKM to manage the symptoms, burdens associated with comorbidities will also remain. Further, the absence of dialysis means that waste products will build up in the patient's blood which might cause other unpleasant symptoms, such as a loss of appetite (Chung *et al.*, 2011).

The most significant removal of burden associated with CKM (aside from the dialysis itself) is a notable reduction in the frequency of visits to an outpatient unit. Given the fact that an elderly patient with significant comorbidities is more likely to be on haemodialysis than peritoneal dialysis,[13] these visits

---

[13]   It is important to note that there is geographical variation in modality, with some countries favouring peritoneal dialysis far more than others.

represent a notable burden for such patients. Depending on the nature of an individual patient's comorbidities it is possible that frequent visits to healthcare facilities will still be necessary, but in general this burden is removed when a patient decides to forego dialysis.

CKM, then, is not a zero-burden option and can still compromise quality of life. It is, however, far less burdensome than dialysis for the average patient. This fact, as I will now discuss, is a key factor in the deliberations of some patients who have the capacity to decide for themselves.

Given the significant burden of dialysis, it is unsurprising that some patients who can decide for themselves choose to forego the treatment even though the alternative – CKM – is in essence an acceptance of death. Understanding the reasons why some patients choose death over dialysis is essential to furthering our understanding of what might be the best option for a patient who lacks decision-making capacity.

Noble and colleagues interviewed capacitous patients in the United Kingdom who chose to forego dialysis, and found commonly occurring reasons for the decision to include: the arduous nature of dialysis; difficulties attending the hospital three times each week; previous knowledge of others on dialysis; and age (Noble *et al.*, 2009). One participant, after describing having witnessed others undergo dialysis, quite definitively asserted that, to his mind, "dead better [sic]".

Similar reasons for choosing CKM over dialysis were echoed in a 2010 systematic review which found that maintaining their current lifestyle was important to patients, with quality of life being prioritised over longevity. Patients gave reasons such as "ability to continue working, maintain a social life, or care for grandchildren" (Morton *et al.*, 2010, p. 6). Whilst in some cases these facts may simply influence treatment modality – i.e. peritoneal dialysis over haemodialysis if possible – in others they lead to the decision to forego dialysis entirely.

It is apparent that quality of life is a major factor in patients' decisions to forego dialysis. The question is, then, what this ought to mean for decisions concerning dialysis for patients who lack decision-making capacity.

3 Bridge therapy

Dialysis has long been a means of maintaining the kidney function of patients awaiting transplantation, acting as a bridge therapy. However, over time dialysis has become more common and is now the first-line treatment for vast numbers of patients (Vandecasteele and Tamura, 2014). It is now more of a lifelong commitment than an interim means of survival for many patients. Whether or not a patient is likely to get a transplant is, therefore, less of a factor in dialysis decisions from a clinical perspective than it once was.

Having already highlighted the ways in which dialysis might be problematic for a patient who lacks decision-making capacity – particularly in terms of potential distress – it follows that putting such a patient through dialysis for the rest of their life is a hugely significant burden. For some such patients a transplant will follow, and this might be considered as justifying the short-term (relative to the remainder of the patient's life) burden of dialysis. For the majority of patients, however, this will not be the case due to the global shortage of organs and the fact that comorbidities may preclude them being deemed good candidates for transplantation.

For those patients who initiate dialysis but for whom a transplant is not a realistic prospect, the question of dialysis discontinuation is likely to arise eventually. Indeed, the only patients for whom it would not arise are those who die whilst on dialysis. Given this, any decision to initiate dialysis when a future transplant is extremely unlikely – or potentially even guaranteed not to happen if the patient is not even deemed eligible to be added to the waiting list – must recognise that withdrawal is inevitable.

It may be more difficult to make the decision to discontinue dialysis than to not initiate it in the first place. Whilst both decisions are recognition that the patient in question is going to die, the latter may not only feel more involved from the point of view of the clinician but also prove complex when discussions must be had with the next-of-kin. Here the equivalence thesis arises. The equivalence thesis is summarised by Wilkinson and Savulescu: "Other things being equal, it is permissible to withdraw a medical treatment that a patient is receiving if it would have been permissible to withhold the same treatment (not already provided), and vice versa" (Wilkinson and Savulescu, 2014, p. 128).

According to the equivalence thesis, there is no moral difference between withholding and withdrawing dialysis assuming all else is equal. Therefore, the question of discontinuation arising ought not to be problematic as withdrawal would only become appropriate if the patient's situation had altered.[14] We know, however, that as much as policies and guidelines employ the equivalence thesis, in practice clinicians *do* acknowledge a difference between withholding and withdrawing (Aberegg *et al.*, 2005). This is attributable to omission bias, whereby clinicians feel that harm caused by action (withdrawal) is worse than harm caused by omission (withholding).

It is problematic if clinicians do perceive the value of continuation to be greater than that of initiation, as in the context of cognitively impaired patients this could mean that a patient remains on dialysis for a significant period of time when it is not appropriate, even if the initiation of dialysis was approp-

---

[14] Arguably, the situation will always have altered to some extent. Indeed – speaking more broadly and not only of dialysis – the purpose of an intervention is generally to change the situation for the better.

riate when that decision was made. The harm this will cause a patient in terms of dialysis burden is disproportionate and thus unacceptable, as well as the fact that the likelihood of that patient experiencing a traumatic event will increase. The initiation of dialysis, then, ought not to act as a delay tactic so that the difficult decision becomes withdrawal rather than initiation. It is important to recognise the equivalence of dialysis withholding and withdrawal to the extent that decisions to withhold or initiate are appropriately made. Then, to dispel omission bias, in later decisions as to the withdrawal of dialysis clinicians – as well as other decision makers – ought to consider the relevance of the doctrine of double effect.

4   Is dialysis worth it?

To subject a patient who cannot consent to the burden of dialysis requires serious thought. In seeking to minimise the harms caused to such a patient, it must be established that the benefits of life extension are sufficient to justify the compromised quality of life.[15] For a significant proportion of patients who lack decision-making capacity, I argue, there is a problematic adherence among decision makers to a vitalism mindset which surfaces in the technological imperative and omission bias.

In questioning the value of life versus death, life is usually concluded to be preferable. This is an understandable default, as not only is life something that we value but also death is irreversible. However, as the worldwide long-term euthanasia debate demonstrates, life is perhaps not something to override all other considerations. There must be a point at which a life-extending intervention is no longer appropriate. If a patient is unable to make their own care decisions, whoever is doing so on their behalf ought to recognise that allowing a patient to die *can* be in their best interests. This is generally understood as the withholding/withdrawal of treatment being in the patient's best interests rather than death itself; death is an acceptable consequence as per the doctrine of double effect.[16] Again, this demonstrates strong negativity surrounding death in many countries.

To conclude that it is sometimes appropriate for patients with or approaching kidney failure who lack decision-making capacity to forego dialysis in favour of CKM, two premises would have to be satisfied:

---

[15]   Even if one approaches it from the other direction, questioning whether the burdens of dialysis are sufficient to justify death, the discussion is equally pertinent.

[16]   This can be seen in the case of *Airedale NHS Trust v Bland 1993* in the United Kingdom, in which the courts did not go so far as to say that Bland's death was in his best interests, but the withdrawal of treatment was.

(a) Where a particular treatment decision is not uncommon among capacitous patients, that same treatment decision must sometimes be appropriate for patients in similar situations who lack decision-making capacity; and

(b) Patients with kidney failure who have decision-making capacity sometimes choose to forego dialysis, instead opting for CKM.

I have already demonstrated (b), so will now turn my attention to (a). Premise (a) speaks to the legal requirements of many countries. The United Nations Convention on the Rights of Persons with Disabilities – currently with 163 signatories – holds that a patient who lacks decision-making capacity ought not to be disadvantaged in the provision of healthcare on the basis of their cognitive impairment (United Nations, 2006). Under the Convention, the mere fact that a patient is cognitively impaired is not grounds to, for instance, withhold treatment. In practice, this means that the purpose of decision making on behalf of a cognitively impaired patient – whatever format that may take in the relevant jurisdiction – is to provide the same care a comparable patient with no cognitive impairment would receive, rather than over- or under-treating, accounting for any known views and/or preferences of the patient in question. This is an important principle to follow, as it seeks to provide equal access to healthcare for the cognitively impaired. Just as it is unfair that such a patient receives a lower quality of care than a capacitous patient, so is it that such a patient receives a higher quality of care. It is about minimising the impact of a patient's cognitive impairment on the entire process of healthcare.

The problem comes in the previously mentioned default of survival. This basic principle of equal treatment regardless of cognitive impairment is ignored when such a patient is dialysed on the basis that living is in everyone's best interests – the technological imperative. It may also be compromised if dialysis is initiated as a default when the deciding party (or parties) is unsure of the best course of action; in Germany (Deutscher Bundestag, 2009, p. 4), as well as in several other countries, the principle of *in dubio pro vita*[17] demonstrates the prevalence of this vitalism mindset.[18]

It is important to recognise that survival is not always preferable, particularly when quality of life is significantly compromised. To action the technological imperative and keep a cognitively impaired patient alive regardless of any compromising of their quality of life is to cause unjustified harm. What I am not suggesting is that because capacitous patients do sometimes forego dialysis that we should *never* dialyze a cognitively impaired patient in case they would too have chosen to forego the intervention. To deny dialysis to the cognitively impaired on the basis of that impairment alone would not only be illegal in most countries but also entirely against the principle of equal access (naturally,

---

[17]   In cases of doubt, the preservation of life is to be favoured.

[18]   It is also ignored if CKM is chosen *because* the patient is cognitively impaired, though this, as discussed, appears to be less of a problem.

it works both ways). Rather, a sometimes-delicate balance must be struck, accounting for the benefits and burdens of each possible course of action as well as any known views and preferences of the patient.

Prevalent in many Western countries, the duty of proportionality requires that doctors achieve care goals through the least restrictive option (Hermerén, 2012). This is important in meeting the demands of non-maleficence, as pursuing anything but the least restrictive option causes unnecessary harm to a patient. CKM is evidently the least restrictive, relative to dialysis. However, care goals vary. For an older cognitively impaired patient the goal of care may be quality of life, which may be achieved through CKM. The care goals for a younger cognitively impaired adult patient may be to allow an active lifestyle which would be better achieved by dialysis (specifically an at-home option if possible). It is, of course, possible that the care goals of a patient are broadly life extension – perhaps based on previously expressed views and preferences – and dialysis may be sought as a result. In such circumstances, however, CKM may still be appropriate depending on the potentially compromised survival benefit of dialysis when a patient has certain comorbidities.

One might argue that the decisions of capacitous patients bear no relation to decisions made on behalf of the cognitively impaired. After all, a patient deciding as to their own care may make a "bad" decision.[19] This is indeed true, and clinicians do have to accept that some patients make decisions which they entirely disagree with, as that is the nature of patient autonomy. It is for this reason that I suggest the fact capacitous patients sometimes forego dialysis ought to mean that patients who lack decision-making capacity ought *sometimes* not to be dialyzed. To truly adhere to the equality of care that is sought for the cognitively impaired, it is important that it reflects the care of those without impairment not only in the availability of options, but also in the decisions made.

5 Conclusion

Decisions concerning dialysis for cognitively impaired patients are not straightforward. A one-off operation with a short recuperation period is likely to more clearly hold value, but dialysis represents a significant long-term burden for (depending on the individual patient) little benefit. I reject the technological imperative and suggest that it can indeed be considered in the best inte-

---

[19] Generally, there is a recognised right to make a "bad" decision afforded to patients. In the United Kingdom, for instance, the Mental Capacity Act 2005 notes that a patient cannot be deemed to lack decision-making capacity on the basis of having made a decision their clinician considers bad. It is for this reason that Jehovah's Witnesses are permitted to refuse blood transfusions.

rests of a cognitively impaired patient to forego dialysis. Many factors are relevant to such a decision, but the fact that some patients do choose CKM suggests that upholding equality in the treatment of the cognitively impaired requires that some do not initiate dialysis.

It is important that any predisposition of clinicians in favour of dialysis does not have an impact on these decisions so that cognitively impaired patients are not subject to disproportionate harm. A tendency towards active treatment may be fuelled by many factors beyond simply the clinician's personal view – a fear of legal action from family, or perhaps business/financial reasons in some health systems – and there is, then, a potential for moral distress (Ducharlet *et al.*, 2019). This is as much an issue as a clinician's personal view guiding a decision, and where this is the case it is important that appropriate measures are put in place to allow clinicians to act in the best interests of patients without feeling constrained by external factors.

My focus has primarily been on the concern of overdialyzing, but underdialyzing is also problematic (MacPhail *et al.*, 2015). The reason for my focus on the former is that it appears to be more prevalent in the literature (Brennan *et al.*, 2017; Clement *et al.*, 2005; Ying *et al.*, 2014). However, it is important to recognise that underdialyzing the cognitively impaired is inevitably an issue to *some extent.*[20] As much as I have outlined reasons why it may be more appropriate for a cognitively impaired patient to begin CKM rather than dialysis, for some dialysis will clearly be the right choice.

Further, I recognise that much of the evidence discussed pertains to elderly patients. This is due to a lack of literature concerning younger adult patients, especially those with cognitive impairments. Given that patients with kidney failure are, on average, elderly, this is unsurprising. It does, however, mean that these perspectives are missing, thereby limiting the applicability of this discussion beyond elderly patients (though it still holds some relevance in a general sense).

In relation to dialysis – and likely many other treatments – further research is needed to better understand the experiences and views of the various parties involved in these complex care decisions. Only then can a more comprehensive picture of the decision-making landscape in the treatment of patients with or approaching kidney failure who lack decision-making capacity be drawn. This is important in developing appropriate guidance for clinicians to aid the decision-making process, ensuring the right decision is made for each patient on an individual basis.

---

[20]   In addition to premature fatalist outlook, clinicians may oppose dialysis for some patients for financial reasons. For instance, less complex patients may be prioritised for dialysis in a pay-for-performance system (Jha *et al.*, 2017). This issue, whilst important, has not been explored in depth as it is applicable only in some countries.

I have demonstrated that the value of dialysis for a cognitively impaired patient is far from clear. The significantly compromised quality of life – reinforced by the fact that this is a key factor in the decisions of capacitous patients to forego dialysis – brings into question the balance of benefits to harms, indicating that starting a patient who lacks decision-making capacity on dialysis might in fact go against the principle of non-maleficence. The question of value is complicated yet further when the patient is not a candidate for eventual transplantation. Where dialysis does not act as a bridge therapy, the patient is being subjected to the burden for the remainder of their life.

The purpose of this chapter has not been to provide an exhaustive discussion of the myriad ethical concerns in the care of cognitively impaired patients with kidney failure, nor a practicable ethical decision-making framework. Rather, I have outlined why dialysis might not be appropriate for a cognitively impaired patient *even if it is life-extending*. The technological imperative – as much as premature fatalism – is a barrier to appropriate care for cognitively impaired patients with or approaching kidney failure, and it is essential that clinicians recognise this and ensure decisions regarding dialysis and CKM are always in the best interests of the patient. Whilst this chapter has focused on kidney failure, parallels can certainly be drawn to decisions on behalf of patients concerning other treatments. Finally, whilst I have been concerned with cognitively impaired patients, many points bear relevance to the care of patients with or approaching kidney failure *with* decision-making capacity.

To close, it is worth briefly touching on the impact the COVID-19 pandemic has had on the issues addressed in this chapter. Whilst this chapter was written prior to the outbreak of the virus, it would be remiss of me not to mention it. First, the pandemic raises ethical issues in kidney care, in part due to the fact that some COVID-19 patients develop acute kidney injuries (Martin *et al.*, 2020; Parsons and Martin, 2020). As with ventilators, there have been concerns that there will be insufficient resources to meet the needs of both long-term patients and those with acute kidney injuries secondary to COVID-19. There is also a fear that patients who are cognitively impaired may be negatively impacted by the additional pressures placed on health systems as they are a vulnerable group (Parsons and Johal, 2020). This is not the place for a detailed discussion of how things are different in present circumstances, but it is important to recognise that they are and that they may continue to be for some time.

References

Aberegg, S. K., Haponik, E. F. and Terry, P. B. (2005), "Omission bias and decision making in pulmonary and critical care medicine", *Chest*, Vol. 128 No. 3, pp. 1497–1505.

Brennan, F., Stewart, C., Burgess, H., Davison, S. N., Moss, A. H., Murtagh, F. E. M., Germain, M., Tranter, S. and Brown, M. (2017), "Time to Improve Informed Consent for Dialysis:

An International Perspective", *Clinical Journal of the American Society of Nephrology*, Vol. 12, pp. 1001–1009.

Chiu, Y. W., Teitelbaum, I., Misra, M., de Leon, E. M., Adzize, T. and Mehrotra, R. (2009), "Pill burden, adherence, hyperphosphatemia, and quality of life in maintenance dialysis patients", *Clinical Journal of the American Society of Nephrology*, Vol. 4 No. 6, pp. 1089–1096.

Chung, S. H., Carrero, J. J. and Lindholm, B. (2011), "Causes of poor appetite in patients on peritoneal dialysis", *Journal of Renal Nutrition*, Vol. 21 No. 1, pp. 12–15.

Clement, R., Chevalet, P., Rodat, O., Ould-Aoudia, V. and Berger, M. (2005), "Withholding or withdrawing dialysis in the elderly: the perspective of a western region of France", *Nephrology Dialysis Transplantation*, Vol. 20, pp. 2446–2452.

Conneen, S., Tzamaloukas, A. H., Adler, K., Keller, L. K., Bordenave, K. and Murata, G. H. (1998), "Withdrawal From Dialysis: Ethical Issues", *Dialysis & Transplantation*, Vol. 27 No. 4, pp. 200–209, 224.

Deutscher Bundestag (2009), *Drucksache 16/13314*.

Ducharlet, K., Philip, J., Gock, H., Brown, M., Gelfand, S. L., Josland, E. A. and Brennan, F. (2019), "Moral Distress in Nephrology: Perceived Barriers to Ethical Clinical Care", *American Journal of Kidney Diseases* [online first].

Findlay, M. D., Dawson, J., Dickie, D. A., Forbes, K. P., McGlynn, D., Quinn, T. and Mark, P. B. (2019), "Investigating the Relationship between Cerebral Blood Flow and Cognitive Function in Hemodialysis Patients", *Journal of the American Society of Nephrology*, Vol. 30 No. 1, pp. 147–158.

Fraser, S. D., Roderick, P. J., May, C. R., McIntyre, N., McIntyre, C., Fluck, R. J., Shardlow, A. and Taal, M. W. (2015), "The burden of comorbidity in people with chronic kidney disease stage 3: a cohort study", *BMC Nephrology*, Vol. 16. No. 193, pp. 1–11.

Fuchs, V. R. (1968), "The growing demand for medical care", *New England Journal of Medicine*, Vol. 279 No. 4, pp. 190–195.

Hermerén, G. (2012), "The principle of proportionality revisited: interpretations and applications", *Medicine, Health Care and Philosophy*, Vol. 15 No. 4, pp. 373–382.

Jha, V., Martin, D. E., Bargman, J. M., Davies, S., Feehally, J., Finkelstein, F., Harris, D., Misra, M., Remuzzi, G., Levin, A. and International Society of Nephrology Ethical Dialysis Task, Force (2017), "Ethical issues in dialysis therapy", *Lancet*, Vol. 389 No. 10081, pp. 1851–1856.

Kaufman, S. R., Shim, J. K. and Russ, A. J. (2006), "Old age, life extension, and the character of medical choice", *Journals of Gerontology. Series B, Psychological Sciences and Social Sciences*, Vol. 61 No. 4, pp. S175–S184.

Li, P. K.-T., Cheung, W. L., Lui, S. L., Blagg, C., Cass, A., Hooi, L. S., Lee, H. Y., Locatelli, F., Wang, T., Yang, C.-W., Canaud, B., Cheng, Y. L., Choong, H. L., de Francisco, A. L., Gura, V., Kaizu, K., Kerr, P. G., Kuok, U. I., Leung, C. B., Lo, W.-K., Misra, M., Szeto, C. C., Tong, K. L., Tungsanga, K., Walker, R., Wong, A. K.-M. and Yu, A. W.-Y. (2011), "Increasing home based dialysis therapies to tackle dialysis burden around the world: A position statement on dialysis economics from the 2nd Congress of the International Society for Hemodialysis", *Nephrology*, Vol. 16 No. 1, pp. 53–56.

MacKillop, E. and Sheard, S. (2018), "Quantifying life: Understanding the history of Quality-Adjusted Life-Years (QALYs)", *Social Science & Medicine*, Vol. 211, pp. 359–366.

MacPhail, A., Ibrahim, J. E., Fetherstonhaugh, D. and Levidiotis, V. (2015), "The Overuse, Underuse, and Misuse of Dialysis in ESKD Patients with Dementia", *Seminars in Dialysis*, Vol. 28 No. 5, pp. 490–496.

Martin, D. E., Parsons, J. A., Caskey, F., Harris, D. C. H. and Jha, V. (2020), "Ethics of kidney care in the era of COVID-19", *Kidney International*, doi: 10.1016/j.kint.2020.09.014

Morton, R. L., Tong, A., Howard, K., Snelling, P. and Webster, A. C. (2010), "The views of patients and carers in treatment decision making for chronic kidney disease: systematic review and thematic synthesis of qualitative studies", *British Medical Journal*, Vol. 340 No. c112, pp. 1–10.

Murtagh, F. E., Marsh, J. E., Donohoe, P., Ekbal, N. J., Sheerin, N. S. and Harris, F. E. (2007), "Dialysis or not? A comparative survival study of patients over 75 years with chronic kidney disease stage 5", *Nephrology Dialysis Transplantation*, Vol. 22 No. 7, pp. 1955–1962.

Nassar, G. M. and Ayus, J. C. (2001), "Infectious complications of the hemodialysis access", *Kidney International*, Vol. 60 No. 1, pp. 1–13.

National Health Service (2018), "Side effects: Dialysis", Available at: https://www.nhs.uk/conditions/dialysis/side-effects/ (accessed 2 December 2020).

National Institute for Health and Care Excellence (2015) "Chronic kidney disease in adults: assessment and management", Clinical Guidance [CG182], Available at: https://www.nice.org.uk/Guidance/CG182 (accessed 2 December 2020).

Noble, H., Meyer, J., Bridges, J., Kelly, D. and Johnson, B. (2009), "Reasons Renal Patients Give for Deciding Not to Dialyze: A Prospective Qualitative Interview Study", *Dialysis & Transplantation*, Vol. 38 No. 3, pp. 82–89.

O'Connor, N. R. and Kumar, P. (2012), "Conservative management of end-stage renal disease without dialysis: a systematic review", *Journal of Palliative Medicine*, Vol. 15 No. 2, pp. 228–235.

O'Dowd, M. A., Jaramillo, J., Dubler, N. and Gomez, M. F. (1998), "A noncompliant patient with fluctuating capacity", *General Hospital Psychiatry*, Vol. 20 No. 5, pp. 317–324.

Parsons, J. A. and Johal, H. K. (2020), "Best interests versus resource allocation: could COVID-19 cloud decision-making for the cognitively impaired?", *Journal of Medical Ethics*, Vol. 46 No. 7, pp. 447–450.

Parsons, J. A. and Martin, D. E. (2020), "A Call for Dialysis-Specific Resource Allocation Guidelines During COVID-19", *American Journal of Bioethics*, Vol. 20 No. 7, pp. 199–201.

Rakowski, D. A., Caillard, S., Agodoa, L. Y. and Abbott, K. C. (2006), "Dementia as a predictor of mortality in dialysis patients", *Clinical Journal of the American Society of Nephrology*, Vol. 1 No. 5, pp. 1000–1005.

Roderick, P., Rayner, H., Tonkin-Crine, S., Okamoto, I., Eyles, C., Leydon, G., Santer, M., Klein, J., Yao, G. L., Murtagh, F., Farrington, K., Caskey, F., Tomson, C., Loud, F., Murphy, E., Elias, R., Greenwood, R. and O'Donoghue, D. (2015), "A national study of practice patterns in UK renal units in the use of dialysis and conservative kidney management to treat people aged 75 years and over with chronic kidney failure", *Health Service Delivery Research*, Vol. 3 No. 12.

Scott, J., Owen-Smith, A., Tonkin-Crine, S., Rayner, H., Roderick, P., Okamoto, I., Leydon, G., Caskey, F. and Methven, S. (2018), "Decision-making for people with dementia and advanced kidney disease: a secondary qualitative analysis of interviews from the Conservative Kidney Management Assessment of Practice Patterns Study", *BMJ Open*, Vol. 8, e022385.

Tagay, S., Kribben, A., Hohenstein, A., Mewes, R. and Senf, W. (2007), "Posttraumatic Stress Disorder in Hemodialysis Patients", *American Journal of Kidney Diseases*, Vol. 50 No. 4, pp. 594–601.

Torres, R. V., Elias, M. F., Seliger, S., Davey, A. and Robbins, M. A. (2017), "Risk for cognitive impairment across 22 measures of cognitive ability in early-stage chronic kidney disease", *Nephrology Dialysis Transplantation*, Vol. 32 No. 2, pp. 299–306.

United Nations (2006), *Convention on the Rights of Persons with Disabilities.*

Vandecasteele, S. J. and Tamura, M. K. (2014), "A Patient-Centered Vision of Care for ESRD: Dialysis as a Bridging Treatment or as a Final Destination?", *Journal of the American Society of Nephrology*, Vol. 25, pp. 1647–1651.

Wilkinson, D. and Savulescu, J. (2014), "A costly separation between withdrawing and withholding treatment in intensive care", *Bioethics*, Vol. 28 No. 3, pp. 127–137.

Ying, I., Levitt, Z. and Jassal, S. V. (2014), "Should an elderly patient with stage V CKD and dementia be started on dialysis?", *Clinical Journal of the American Society of Nephrology*, Vol. 9 No. 5, pp. 971–977.

Contributors

Karla Alex holds a graduate degree in Philosophy and German Studies from Heidelberg University and studied in Heidelberg, Berlin, Bamberg, and Lexington (KY). She specialized in applied ethics, especially medical ethics, and in modern German literature studies, especially the work of Rainer Maria Rilke. She is currently working as a research associate at Heidelberg University Hospital as part of the philosophical subproject of the DFG funded project "Comparative Assessment of Genome and Epigenome Editing in Medicine: Ethical, Legal and Social Implications" (COMPASS-ELSI). Within medical ethics, she is particularly interested in ethical questions at the beginning and end of life as well as in connection with legal issues.

Charlotte Buch is a researcher at the Institute for History and Ethics of Medicine at the Martin Luther University Halle-Wittenberg. She has studied Business Administration in Mannheim (University of Mannheim) and Seoul, South Korea (Sogang University), and health economics (University of Bayreuth). Her research interests include ethical questions of digitalization in health care, ethics and health economics, and hospital management.

Sebastian Himmler is health economics PhD candidate at the Erasmus School of Health Policy & Management In Rotterdam. He is applying economic and statistical tools, including applied econometrics, health economic modelling, and discrete choice experiments, to conduct research on topics surrounding the efficient allocation of health care resources. He is a health economist by training (University of Bayreuth), with research stays in the United States (UNC Chapel Hill) and Denmark (SDU Odense), and part of a European PhD training network ("Improving Quality of Care in Europe").

Paul Mark Mitchell is a Research Fellow in Health Economics at the University of Bristol in the UK. He has over a decade of experience working on the capability approach, that was initially developed by Amartya Sen. He is a coordinator for the health and disability thematic group for the Human Development and Capability Association. He obtained his PhD in Health Economics at the University of Birmingham, UK. He also studied at the National University of Ireland, Galway, at masters (Economic Policy Evaluation and Planning) and undergraduate (Commerce) levels.

Karolina Napiwodzka is a PhD candidate at Chair of Ethics, Faculty of Philosophy of Adam Mickiewicz University in Poznań, Poland. Her doctoral dissertation concerns the relations between doctors and patients in the light of Jürgen Habermas' discourse theory. She is mainly interested in philosophy of medicine, medical ethics and communication in medicine.

Jordan A. Parsons is a PhD candidate at the Centre for Ethics in Medicine at the University of Bristol, UK. His research is funded by the Wellcome Trust through the BABEL project (Balancing Best Interests in Healthcare Ethics and Law) and explores best interests decision making in the context of kidney failure. Jordan's background is in politics and philosophy, and his research interests include ethical issues in kidney care, transplantation, reproductive health, and genetics.

Jan Schildmann is a specialist in internal medicine and director of the Institute for History and Ethics of Medicine at the Martin Luther University Halle-Wittenberg. He has studied medicine and holds postgraduate degrees in medical law and ethics (King' College London) and philosophy (Fernuniversität Hagen). His research interests cover a broad spectrum of topics in clinical as well as research ethics.

Petra Schnell-Inderst is a Senior Scientist and Head of the Program on Health Technology Assessment (HTA) at the Department of Public Health, Health Services Research and HTA at UMIT – University for Health Sciences, Medical Informatics and Technology in Hall i. T., Austria. She is the Institute's Representative for the European Network for Health Technology Assessment. After her studies in Biology (Dipl.-Biol.), she specialised in Epidemiology and Public Health (MPH) at the Ludwig-Maximilians-University Munich. Her main research interests are in health technology assessment methodology with a focus on medical devices, digital health technologies, personalised cancer medicine, and public health interventions.

Uwe Siebert is Professor of Public Health, Medical Decision Making and Health Technology Assessment (UMIT), Chair of the Dept. of Public Health, Health Services Research and HTA at UMIT, and Adjunct Professor of Health Policy and Management at the Harvard Chan School of Public Health. His research interests include applying evidence-based and translational methods from public health and medicine in the framework of medical decision making, patient guidance and HTA. He is Past-President of the Society for Medical Decision Making (SMDM) and member of several boards of directors of scientific associations.

Caroline Steigenberger is a Junior Scientist at the Program on Health Technology Assessment (HTA) at the Department of Public Health, Health Services Research and HTA at UMIT – University for Health Sciences, Medical Informatics and Technology in Hall i. T., Austria. She is currently enrolled in the doctoral programme (Dr.phil.) in Public Health at UMIT. She studied Health Economics at the Fresenius University of Applied Sciences and received a Master of Public Health (MPH) from the Ludwig-Maximilians-University Munich in 2015. Her research interests cover a broad spectrum in the area of medical decision making, patient-orientation in health care, and health economic evaluation.

Francisca Stutzin Donoso is a clinical psychologist from Santiago, Chile. She holds postgraduate degrees in contemporary thought (Diego Portales University), philosophy, politics and economics of health (University College London) and she is completing a PhD in health humanities (University College London, Health Humanities Centre). Her research focuses on health outcomes inequalities for chronic diseases, long-term treatment adherence and the lived experience of chronic diseases.

Jasper Ubels is a doctoral student in health economics at the German Cancer Research Centre (DKFZ) and the Mannheim Medical Faculty of the University of Heidelberg. He completed his Master of Science in Public Health with a specialisation in Health Economics at Umeå University, Sweden. For his dissertation, he studies how the capability approach can be applied to assess the value of medical interventions.

Jürgen Zerth is Professor for Economics, especially Health Economics at Wilhelm Loehe University for Applied Science and Head of Research Institute IDC, both located in Fuerth. He studied economics and health economics at Universities in Bamberg and Bayreuth. Zerth was Interim Professor at Friedrich-Alexander-University Erlangen-Nuremberg and Visiting Lecturer at Shanghai International Studies University, China. His research topics of interest are health economics and health policy, economics in long-term care and management strategies for care and cure organizations.